CONVERSATIONS

ON *Health & Wellness*

Insight Publishing
Sevierville, Tennessee

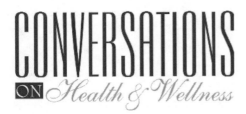

CONVERSATIONS
ON *Health & Wellness*

© 2004 by Insight Publishing Company.

Published by Insight Publishing Company
P.O. Box 4189
Sevierville, Tennessee 37864

10 9 8 7 6 5 4 3 2

Printed in the United States of America

ISBN: 1-932863-07-9

Table Of Contents

A Message From The Publisher

This book is more than a collection of interviews from men and women who care about your health and well being. *Conversations on Health and Wellness* is an intimate introduction into the lives and hearts of seventeen very special people, people who are passionate about living and living well! Each contributor has a story that deserves to be told. Through their stories, and the lessons they've learned, you can discover new insights into your own physical and emotional health.

I've learned that advice from a trusted friend with whom you have a shared experience is usually advice worth considering. The woman fighting chronic pain can trust a friend who is battling the same demons and who recently discovered a therapy that helps. A daughter with cancer can find comfort from her mom, a cancer survivor. The overweight man struggling to improve his health through diet and exercise is open to the counsel from a close friend who has lost 50 pounds and kept off the weight.

I hope you'll consider these professionals trustworthy advisors. Their insights and strategies deserve careful consideration. If something they recommend sounds reasonable and might help you improve your health, I hope you will talk to those whom you trust and consider implementing their ideas.

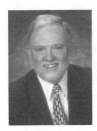

Interviews conducted by:

David E. Wright
President, International Speakers Network

Chapter 1

REBECCA HULEM, RN, RNP, CNM
CERTIFIED MENOPAUSE CLINICIAN

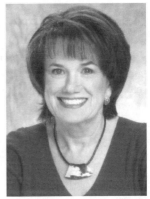

THE INTERVIEW

David E. Wright (Wright)

Here with Rebecca Hulem, for over twenty eight years Rebecca has shared her knowledge, experience and expertise in the field of women's health. Early in her career, she worked as a registered nurse in labor and delivery. Her passion for learning and desire to be of greater service to women took her back to school to become an OB-GYN nurse practitioner and certified nurse midwife. While working as a nurse midwife, Rebecca delivered over two thousand babies. It was during her own transition through menopause and the difficulties she encountered with the symptoms of menopause, that fueled her passion to become a certified menopause clinician. In 2003, Rebecca left the cozy corporate world to start her own business as a speaker and author. She has traveled throughout the United States and Canada, speaking to professional nurses and lay women about the many aspects of menopause. Her first book, *Feelin' Hot?*, A Humorous, Informative and Truthful Look at Menopause, has been a great success and is now in it's second printing. Rebecca welcome to *Conversations on Health and Wellness.*

Rebecca Hulem (Hulem)

Thank you David, it is a pleasure to be here.

Wright

Tell me a little bit about your background, and why you have become so passionate about helping women through menopause.

Hulem

As you mentioned in my introduction, I have spent over twenty eight years of my career working with women, of all ages and in all stages of their life. I have had the opportunity to counsel young girls going through puberty and having difficulty with their menstrual periods. I've followed women through their pregnancies and had the privilege of delivering their babies, and most recently have started to specialize in women who are in some phase of menopause. When I went through menopause myself and I realized how difficult a transformation it can be, I decided I really wanted to focus my attention more specifically on women going through menopause, as opposed to women across the life span.

Wright

From your book, *Feelin' Hot?*, you appear to have a unique approach to dealing with menopause. Could you tell us what is your philosophy, and how did this evolve for you.

Hulem

My philosophy, David, is that every woman is a very unique individual. Even though women will have similar symptoms when they go through menopause such as hot flashes, night sweats, sleep disturbances, and mood swings I believe it is very important that we, meaning the medical community, media, and consumer products industry, stop trying to treat every single woman exactly the same as we have for decades. For close to fifty years we have advocated that every woman should take hormones to treat these symptoms. It's similar to a "one size fits all" mentality. It is my belief that every woman needs to be looked at as an individual and looked at in terms of what's going on with her body, as an individual and what can we offer her to help her feel better without putting her at risk for long term disease. Up until recently, the medical community, in my opinion, has taken a very simplistic approach, by offering the same solution to every woman, but fortunately what we've learned over time, is that it doesn't work for every woman, we have to really look at them individually and say, "OK, what will best help this woman."

Wright

You know I have had some experience with the uniqueness of women, my wife and I had been married twelve years, she was thirty eight years old, and she started going through early menopause. Even before that, the infertility experts had said she would never bear children, so we didn't even think about it. When we got married we had decided that it wasn't that important that we have children. At thirty nine she had her first child!

Hulem

Surprise!!

Wright

Now, that's kind of strange, I thought you couldn't have children after you went through menopause.

Hulem

Well, generally, you can't. Your situation sounds like a perfect example of how confusing it can be for women when they start the transition into menopause, which is called perimenopause. This transition can start to occur as early as mid to late thirties and when this happens, for the most part, the ovary, which is the organ that produces a ripened egg every month, is starting to shut down. When this occurs a woman's menstrual periods will not come on a regular basis. She may go for months without a period. This is where the confusion comes in because as women we have been taught that if we're not having regular periods then we can't get pregnant. But until a woman goes one full year without a menstrual period she is not considered to be finished with menopause. Every once in a while, the ovary can kick out one more egg, and then surprise there you go, you have a baby! So this can be a very confusing time for women.

Wright

Well, I'm so glad that it happened.

Hulem

I bet you are!

3

Wright

I have a fifteen year old to prove it!

Hulem

Aren't you a lucky man? If you have a daughter you better save your money. She's probably thinking about having her own car around this time. And then there is the prom, college, and maybe a wedding.

Wright

You know many women describe themselves, as feeling crazy, while transitioning through menopause. What's that all about?

Hulem

The feeling crazy comes from hormonal fluctuations that are starting to happen during the perimenopause period of the menopause transition. The level of three very important hormones, estrogen, progesterone and testosterone that have been produced in abundance ever since the woman went through puberty, are starting to fluctuate now. So the body isn't producing the same amount of hormones, and with a decline of these hormones comes a lot of different symptoms. For example "fuzzy thinking" is a big complaint among women who are going through perimenopause. This is when they can't quite remember the word that they want to use to describe what they are trying to say. Or they will become easily distracted and walk into a room and can't remember why they walked in there. Hormone fluctuation can cause a lot of these symptoms.

Another symptom that women experience from hormone fluctuation is mood swings. When a woman is having mood swings it is usually caused from a decline in the hormone progesterone. Progesterone is produced by the ovary during ovulation. When the level of progesterone begins to decline during perimenopause she may get easily frustrated and start to lose her patience, and this situation is very disturbing for women because women are relationship oriented, we thrive on the relationships we build throughout our life, and when we lose our patience and are moody and snap at the people we love, we feel out of control and this makes us feel like we are loosing our mind.

Wright

So we know that menopause affects how women feel physically and emotionally. Will this have an impact on the people around them, such as their life partner, their children or even the people that they work with?

Hulem

Oh, yes, menopause will affect just about everybody because when you stop and think about it, just in the United States alone, there's fifty million women going through some stage of menopause. Now these fifty million women are probably working so they have co-workers and colleagues, and the symptoms we are talking about don't just occur when a woman is at home. She may be having hot flashes, mood swings and fuzzy thinking at work, which may affect her pro-ductivity, which in turn will affect her coworkers and colleagues. The majority of women are generally married or have a partner, and when they start having these mood changes , night sweats ,hot flashes or they can't remember where they put their car keys, this will affect their relationship with their partner as well.

Another situation that has a tremendous impact on a woman's re-lationship with her partner is that many women, when they go through menopause, lose their desire to have sex. If this happens their partners get very confused and they think, "What happened?" Men feel rejected, when a woman doesn't show the same amount of affection and love to them, as they once did and yet they feel uncom-fortable asking, "What's going on"? If a woman has teenagers while she is going through perimenopause and menopause this can be a whole different challenge for both the woman and the teenager. For example we all know that teenagers have unique ways of getting their needs met, which can be a little manipulating at times. When a woman is feeling like herself she can deal with the challenges that having a teenager in the house brings, but when a woman isn't feel-ing good, and she is having these mood swings and she's not sleeping and she's tired, she just can't put up with the shenanigans that teen-agers pull, so then all the sudden the teenager thinks, " Oh my gosh my mother is going crazy, she can't remember from one day to the next what I told her, she's grumpy all the time," so yes menopause will have an affect on just about everybody around you.

Wright

Other than the symptoms of hot flashes, night sweats, mood changes and sleep disturbances, are there any significant health risks during or after menopause that women should be aware of?

Hulem

Yes, there are several different health risks; one most importantly is heart disease. What many women don't understand and don't really know, mainly because the media and medical community have put so much emphasis on breast cancer, is that heart disease will actually kill one out of every two women, over the age of fifty.

Wright

WOW!

Hulem

The reality is there is only a four percent lifetime risk of dying from breast cancer, but there is a fifty percent lifetime risk of dying from heart disease. The other significant health risk is osteoporosis. Women also have a 50% chance of having a fracture of their hip, spine, wrist, or ankle caused by osteoporosis. Again we have put a lot of emphasis on breast cancer and this isn't to say that reducing the incidence of breast cancer is not important, it most certainly is but we also need to educate women on the best ways to protect themselves from loss of bone as they age. We need to start this education early in a woman's life. As early as her teenage years when her bones start really developing their strength and integrity and then continue the education through out her adult years. This will give her more control over the out come. This education should include not only eating well and taking calcium, but also, doing some form of weight bearing exercise, throughout her adult years. Other long term health concerns that can occur during menopause or beyond, is if a woman is over weight, she's more prone to developing diabetes and if she develops diabetes, this will put her at greater risk for heart disease and stroke. Many studies are showing that if a woman is over weight she is also at a greater risk for developing cancer.

Wright

Wow! You know there's so much controversy surrounding hormone replacement therapy, since the Women's Health Initiative study was released in 2002. What is your opinion about hormones?

Hulem

Well my opinion is based on two things, my professional experience, certainly, and also my personal experience with hormones. Hormones given to women while they are going through menopause can be very effective, as long as women understand that they are not to be taken for the rest of their life. Now this is different from what we used to say, prior to the Women's Health Initiative study. We used to recommend to women that they begin taking hormones at the start of menopause, and plan on taking them for the rest of their life.

This recommendation was based on the belief that there were more benefits to taking hormones than there were risks. For example, we thought it would help protect them from heart disease, but what we found out, from the Women's Health Initiative study, was not only does it not protect against heart disease, but in fact, it may put many women at greater risk for heart attacks and stroke. Some women will need to take hormones initially in the early years of menopause, to help alleviate the most bothersome symptoms, such as hot flashes, night sweats and mood swings. Early years, meaning the first three to five years that they go through menopause. When given during this time period, I think for most women they are probably safe. Studies have consistently shown that when women are on hormones longer than a 5-10 year period, significant health problems can start to show up. Such as a greater incidence of breast cancer, heart attack and stroke. I sincerely believe that women need to have a stronger reliance on healthy lifestyle choices such as healthy eating, daily exercise and vitamin supplementation, as opposed to relying on hormones as the magic pill. The medical community needs to make this a bigger priority in the health care system as well.

Wright

Do you think all women should take hormones?

Hulem

Not necessarily. This is where individualizing a woman's health care is so important. I think that there's only a small category of women that will need to take hormones. For example, now the only reason why a woman would decide to take hormones is because she is having symptoms that are impacting her day to day quality of life. If she's having hot flashes every ten minutes or she is awake every ten minutes at night with night sweats, or she is so moody that she's been told to go away and don't come back until she gets her moods under control, these are all good reasons to consider hormone therapy. And this will be a very small percentage of women, approximately forty percent of women that really need to take hormones. The other sixty percent of women may choose not to take hormones and instead will want to try alternatives to hormones, like herbs, vitamins, or dietary supplements for their symptoms. And out of this same remaining sixty percent believe it or not there will be some women who won't need to take anything at all except to change their eating habits or include exercise in their daily lives because their symptoms aren't really that significant. So every woman, again, needs to be looked at and treated as an individual, and not one size fits all.

Wright

So, let me see if I understand you correctly, there will be situations where women could change their eating habits and maybe exercise more and that would do the same thing as hormonal treatments?

Hulem

In some regards it will, as long as the symptoms aren't too severe. For example, if a woman is exercising regularly, that's going to make her feel well in so many ways. Exercise increases the circulation throughout the body, and it increases serotonin levels in the brain, so it gives the woman a greater since of well being. Studies have shown that women, who exercise regularly, do have fewer hot flashes than women who don't. It also helps them to control their weight, and weight is a big issue for most women. We never feel that we are thin enough, and particularly when we go through menopause and our metabolism slows down, we tend to gain weight a lot easier than we did when we were, say, in our thirties. So exercise will help control her weight, she'll look better in her clothes, so she'll feel better about herself. Exercise also helps a woman sleep better. So exercise can accomplish a lot of things, that hormones do as well, but it is just a healthier way to go.

Wright

Is there an average length of time that you think women can safely take hormones?

Hulem

I believe women can safely take hormones for about five years. Now certainly this is an individual thing. Many women have been on hormones for twenty years or longer and have no significant health problems. There is always going to be an exception to every rule. But aging is hard on the body and our bodies need all the care and attention we can give them to keep us going throughout our life. I strongly believe that healthy eating which includes an abundance of fruits, vegetables, fiber, and plant based proteins in a diet as well as regular exercise will keep us all healthy longer than any hormone we can possibly take. I suggest to my patients that after five years of taking hormones we need to reconsider their individual situation and take a look at, how are they feeling? Why are they taking the hormones? Do they have good lifestyle choices in place, like healthy eating and exercising. And then if that's the case then try to reduce the dosage, the amount of hormones they are taking or the number of days of the week that they are taking them, and see if they can do well without them.

I believe it is my job as their health care provider to encourage healthy lifestyle choices and help them develop these healthy habits in addition to prescribing hormones. Now some women are going to be on hormones for ten or twenty years, and other women may be on hormones for two years. Every woman is going to be a little bit different. There are so many variables to take in to consideration when developing a health plan for each woman. But I would like to see us get away from taking hormones as a lifetime regimen.

Wright

The hormones that were used in the Women's Health Initiative study were synthetic, commercially produced hormones, what do women mean when they talk about natural bio-identical compounded hormones?

Hulem

Natural bio-identical compounded hormones are different from synthetic commercially produced hormones in several ways. The first difference is that bio-identical compounded hormones are not mass produced or commercially produced in large quantities. A prescription for bio-identical compounded hormones must be taken to a pharmacy that specializes in compounding medications. So for example, you wouldn't be able to get a prescription for bio-identical compounded hormones filled at your local Sav-On or Rite-Aide pharmacy because these pharmacies don't make up compounded medications. The second way that bio-identical hormones are different from synthetic hormones is in the molecular structure of the hormone. In synthetic hormones produced by a large pharmaceutical company the molecular structure of the hormone has been changed slightly from how it is found in the body. The pharmaceutical company that makes commercially made hormones are required by the FDA to change the molecular structure in order to be issued a patent on the hormone. Bio-identical hormones are not FDA approved, they are not patented, and therefore the molecular structure of the hormone is still in its natural state as it would normally be found in a woman's body.

The advantage to putting a molecularly identical hormone into a woman's body is that the body readily identifies it as something it knows and is familiar with. This way it can then utilize it easily, thereby creating fewer and sometimes no side effects. The disadvantages to prescribing bio-identical hormones is that because they are not FDA approved many times insurance companies will not cover the cost of these hormones. They can be very expensive because they are individually made for each woman and then this cost has to be absorbed by the woman herself. Another disadvantage is that because they are not FDA approved there aren't the large clinical trials available on their safety or efficacy as with synthetic hormones so we don't really know if they are safer. Until there are more studies done on bio-identical hormones and we have more answers to their safety we have to assume that they carry the exact same risk to women as synthetic hormones do, even though they may produce fewer side effects.

Wright

If women don't want to or can't take hormones, are there any safe alternatives that will relieve their symptoms and help them through this phase in their life?

Hulem

Yes, there are many alternatives that are out on the market now, for example, some women are turning to herbs and the most common herb is called Black Cohosh. Black Cohosh has been around and been used extensively for decades in Germany, for women that are having hot flashes and women that are having mood swings. And we have brought it here in the states probably within the last five to ten years. There is a commercially made Black Cohosh, which is called Remifemin and this is the most standardized form of Black Cohosh and generally considered the safest form of this particular herb. Black Cohosh is usually taken twice a day and its main purpose is to relieve hot flashes and mood swings. There are other herbs that are on the market, as well as soy products. Soy has become very popular in the United States. For centuries Japanese women have been eating soy in their diet and Japanese women don't even have a word for hot flashes, and researchers are beginning to feel that is because of the soy. Soy actually has a weak estrogenic affect in a woman's body. Estrogen is the hormone that is responsible for regulating our body temperature. So many women here in the United States and around the world are now turning to soy to help them relieve their hot flashes. There's also things like aromatherapy essential oils, which have been used for mood swings and help calm and relax the body and mind.

So there are many things that women can use instead of hormones. I generally recommend that if a woman wants to use herbs or alternative methods that they go to a naturopathic physician or they go to an herbalist who has been trained in prescribing these herbs or alternatives, and that way they have a medical person that they can consult with and that can guide them along, rather than just going out to the local health food store and buying the first thing that they see on the shelf.

Wright

Let me see if I can connect some dots here. Do you mind?

Hulem

Not at all.

Wright

So hormones are naturally produced by a healthy body.

Hulem

Correct.

Wright

Once something happens and these hormones are not being produced, there are synthetic or commercially produced hormones as well as bio-identical compounded hormones that could be prescribed and given to a woman that would actually replace the ones that the body is no longer producing. Is that correct?

Hulem

That's correct. And it is also important to know there is a difference between synthetic and bio-identical compounded hormones, just by the way that they are made, but they are both hormones.

Wright

But they are both hormones?

Hulem

Yes, Synthetic hormones are FDA approved, bio-identical hormones have not been FDA approved, but they have similar benefits and as far as we know, the same risks.

Wright

So then the third option to treat the symptoms, would be through herbs, and alternatives, something other than hormones

Hulem

That's correct.

Wright

Something from a health food store.

Hulem

Or a woman can be given herbs or dietary supplements from a Naturopath physician or an herbalist who specializes in dispensing herbs for certain medical conditions. I think this is a better choice than just buying an herb or dietary supplement over the counter. This way a woman has a trained professional who is following her and can guide her if she is having any reaction to the herb or supplement. If she just buys it over the counter and she experiences side effects or problems, who is she going to go to? The clerk at the health food store probably won't know what to tell her other than to sell her another product.

Wright

So for example, if the lack of the hormones created the night sweats and a woman goes to a naturopath physician or an herbalist and gets an herb but she is still having night sweats she can then go back to the physician and discuss that she is still having problems and together they can figure out a solution? But the important point to make here is that there are many choices other than hormones that are available to take away the symptoms of menopause.

Hulem

That's correct David. There are many women and many choices. Each woman should be given the education about her choices and the right to explore the choices that are best for her.

Wright

Ok, I am beginning to understand it.

Hulem

Now you know why it can be so confusing to women. There are so many choices available to women today. And this particular area of medicine is changing so quickly it's hard to keep up with. Plus women receive so many mixed messages from the media, magazines, and the medical community they don't know which way to turn. This is why women really need education about this particular phase of life, and they need to understand how their body works. Even though we learned this in our biology class in high school we quickly forgot it and went on with our life, unless of course you go into the medical field then you know it extensively.

I think women should be offered a class when they start into menopause, something similar to the prepared childbirth classes that are offered to couples when they are going to have a baby. I feel so strongly about the need for education that I started a class called: Sexy, Serene and Self Assured: The New Guide to Menopause. The majority of women don't pay that much attention to their body or how it works, they just take it for granted that it is going to continue working the way it always has. When things start to change as early as their late thirties they are caught by surprise. This class has been a tremendous success. If women have partners they are welcome to bring their partners to class also. This way both parties have an understanding as to what is going on. I explain step by step what is happening in a woman's body, the difference and importance between all three hormones that were once produced by a woman's ovaries and what hormone is responsible for what symptom. I go over the benefits and risks of taking hormones, and the many different kinds of hormones that are available, their similarities and their differences.

Many women aren't aware that not only are there many different types of hormones available, there are also many different ways to take hormones other than by pill form. For example a woman can take hormones by pills, patches, creams, and vaginal rings. Many women don't know this nor do they know the benefits of taking hormones in a different form. I also explain what alternatives to hormones are available and what the benefit is to using an alternative other than a hormone. We also discuss sexual changes and how it will affect both parties.

Wright

During menopause, you mentioned earlier there is a possibility that a woman will lose her desire for sex. Would that be a mental condition, brought on by lack of hormones? Surely it couldn't be a physical condition, could it?

Hulem

Well you know this is an excellent question David, I'm glad you brought this up because actually, a decreased desire for sex during menopause is both physical and mental. The physical part of it is caused by two hormones, estrogen and testosterone. Testosterone used to be produced by a woman's ovaries during her ovulation cycles. You know about testosterone because that is the main sex hormone that you have in your body, but women don't have nearly as much testosterone as men do. But they do have a little bit, and it's produced by their ovaries and is also produced by their adrenal glands. The purpose of the testosterone is to give the woman a desire to have sex. Mother Nature designed it so that when a woman ovulated and produced an egg, testosterone was produced at the same time. And it makes sense that if you're ovulating, you've got an egg and this is the best time for you to get pregnant, that you also have to have the desire, so mother nature gave a woman testosterone and the testosterone gave her the desire to have sex. So if she had sex and she wasn't using birth control, she would generally get pregnant. But when you go through menopause, the body says, well you're in your fifties, there' s probably no real reason why you would want to continue on and have babies at this point in your life, so everything shuts down and the testosterone that the ovaries used to produce shuts down as well.

Another hormone that is produced by the ovary is estrogen. Estrogen does many wonderful things for a woman's body and it affects just about every organ system a woman has. The way estrogen relates to sex is without a steady supply of estrogen a woman will no longer have lubrication in the vagina, and without lubrication in the vagina intercourse will become very painful. So now a woman is no longer producing any where near the level of testosterone as she used to when she was in her twenties and thirties, so she looses the desire to have sex, and without enough estrogen it hurts to have sex. To complicate matters further from a mental or an emotional stand point, if she's not getting enough sleep, she is probably tired. If she is tired then she is going to be moody and if she is moody, then the last thing she is going to want to do is have sex. A woman's mind and body doesn't think, nor work the way a man's does. We have to be in the mood.

Wright

I've noticed!

Hulem

So, yes testosterone is a big key for lack of desire for a woman going through menopause, but women also need to know, that while these hormones are fluctuating and they are experiencing all these symptoms, this situation won't last forever. Most of the symptoms will eventually go away. As the body regains its equilibrium she will emerge into a new woman. Now her desire for sex will probably not ever be as ravenous as when she was in her twenties or thirties, but it will still come back somewhat, she still will be able and want to have intimacy with her partner, for a long time to come. It's just that during this period of time it can be a little upsetting and challenging for both the woman and the man.

Wright

Before I ask you the last question, I've got another question this past discussion has brought on. Is there anything that a man can do? The number one thing I imagine is just realizing the problems of menopause. After I've discussed this with you over the last thirty minutes, it occurred to me that the most important thing I can do is understand what a woman is going through.

Hulem

You're absolutely right David

Wright

But beyond that, is there anything I can do, that would facilitate more of a sex drive?

Hulem

I recommend to husbands and partners of women who are going through menopause, to first understand that it's a natural process that a woman's body goes through and that it not only affects her physically, but it will affect her emotionally and mentally as well. If they understand this is a temporary process that the woman's body naturally has to go through, then they also won't take it personally. And it is very important that a man does not take a women's lack of a desire for sex personally because it really has nothing to do with not loving him or not wanting to be with him. So what a man can do is perhaps take on the role of the initiator during this period of time, but with the thought in mind, what do you need from me, what can I do to help make this pleasurable for both of us, and make this exciting for both of us. And if a man can just go back to the basics, for example, when you were dating your wife, you made special arrangements to take her out to a nice restaurant, to a movie or to take her to a play. You paid attention to her; you took the time to listen to her and asked her how she was feeling. You had a genuine concern for her welfare as your partner. What you can do to help her is to remind her that you do understand and that you want to help her through this. And that this is something that both of you are going through and that you don't want her to feel alone.

Wright

That is good advice. Right now I have two friends, co-workers, in two separate industries that have both just gotten divorces, and said their marriages were unpleasant or whatever, but now that they have met someone new it is almost like they are teenagers again. And so I am thinking, and forgive me for being a man, but wait a minute, why didn't you make it that exciting for the husband that you just divorced, and maybe you would not have had to go through that.

Hulem

That's a reasonable assumption, but researchers have actually done studies and found that you can take a woman in menopause that has no sexual desire and put her with a new partner or a younger new partner and until the honeymoon phase of the relationship is over, she will be just as excited and just as ready to go as she was when she was with her previous partner. But then once all the excitement wears off, she may lose her desire again. See what we tend to do in relationships? We tend to become very complacent, particularly when we have been with someone for a long time. You know we all get into our habits and we just don't try as hard anymore, we don't try to make the relationship exciting. We start taking each other for granted and then we just expect that the other person should and wants to fulfill all of our needs. So communication is the most important thing for couples to always keep open, but particularly during the time when a woman's going through these physical changes that she really has no control over. This is just what her body does and it would be no different if you were having a male menopause. In fact many people have asked, is there a male menopause? And there is somewhat of a male menopause but it doesn't seem to be as dramatic, physically for a man as it does for a woman and if it does become more physically dramatic, now they have Viagra for men. We don't yet have the same types of drugs to give a woman that will elicit the same type of response as Viagra does for men. Scientists are trying to come up with something, but for now women are left to hoping that they can communicate with their partners about what's going on so their partners will understand and with the understanding they will find other ways to get their sexual needs met.

The other thing that men need to understand too is that with a woman's body, not only does she lose the desire, but her body may not respond to the same stimulus as when she was younger. When her body isn't responding men again tend to think, well she's not interested, she doesn't care or she doesn't find me attractive anymore. So it may take longer to make love and achieve the level of satisfaction each of you are looking for, but with good communication and the willingness to explore new ways of making love each partner can continue to feel loved and intimacy will continue to grow in the relationship.

Wright

Well, very, very interesting. Let me ask you a final question, what do you think is the best way for a woman to prepare for menopause?

Hulem

I think the best way is certainly through education. I want to see women and men become educated on this phase of life, long before they ever reach it. We need to start thinking about it in our late thirties and early forties as opposed to waiting to our fifties, when all the sudden it just comes on us like a freight train. So women need to be educated about this time of life and what to expect, either by reading or taking classes through her local hospital. Many times health care providers have courses on this subject. I am hoping that some day this course will be offered in community colleges, and made available for women and men to take, either together or separately. So educate yourself on this phase of life and try not to be afraid of it because even though, yes, it's a physical change, and ok so it says we are not getting any younger, but we are getting a little older, things are slowing down and things are going to be different, it's still a wonderful stage of life, and we have so much more to look forward to.

Statistics have shown that once a woman turns fifty, she will probably have another thirty, forty or even fifty years to live, so there's a lot that can be accomplished. I never dreamed that I would write a book or be speaking all over the world after I went through menopause. We can't possibly know what life has in store for us throughout our lives. I also think that it is important for women to remember while preparing for this stage, that it's not just physical changes that they need to address. Our mind, body and spirit are all one entity. Everything really is connected. If you look at it through a holistic point of view, and ask yourself how can I solve the physical problems but also stay connected to family, friends and the community and how can I reduce the stress in my life, either by exercising regularly ,eating well, maybe taking meditation classes, yoga classes, something that is going to help relax my mind and my body and bring the spiritual connection back into my life, you will probably not only live longer, but will live in a healthier state all the days of your life.

Wright

Well, what an entertaining conversation, I have really learned a lot, I wish I would have talked to you twenty-five years ago.

Hulem

You know a lot of people say that. That's why I'm so passionate about this subject and this very special time in life. I want to get this information out into the world so we can improve the quality of our lives.

Wright

I understand that. Today we have been talking to Rebecca Hulem, for over twenty-eight years she has shared her knowledge and expertise in the field of women's health, she travels throughout the United States and Canada speaking to professional nurses and lay women about the many aspects of menopause. As we have found here today she knows quite a bit about it. Rebecca, I really do appreciate you spending so much time with me today and it's just been a pleasure talking with you on *Conversations on Health and Wellness*.

Hulem

Thank you, David; it's been my pleasure, as well.

About The Author

Rebecca Hulem has excelled in the field of women's health for over twenty-eight years. Her career has included positions as a registered nurse, Ob/Gyn nurse practitioner, certified menopause clinician, and certified nurse midwife. Along the way, Rebecca has personally delivered over two thousand babies.

In 2003, Rebecca left the corporate world to start her own business as a dynamic speaker and author on the subject of menopause. She has traveled throughout the Untied States and Canada speaking professionally to women of all ages on how to stay healthy and sane in spite of their hormones. Her first book, *Feelin' Hot?* A Humorous, Informative and Truthful Look at Menopause is now in its second printing.

Rebecca Hulem, RN, RNP, CNM

"The Menopause Expert"

5737 Kanan Road #261

Agoura Hills, California 91301-1601

Phone: 818-889-2475 #2

FAX: 818-991-3570

E-Mail: Rebecca@themenopauseexpert.com

www.themenopauseexpert.com

Chapter 2

DR. JOHN GRAY

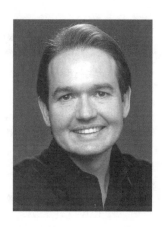

THE INTERVIEW

David E. Wright (Wright)

We are talking to Doctor John Gray. Dr. Gray is a Certified Family Therapist, Consulting Editor of the *Family Journal*, a member of the Distinguished Advisory Board of the International Association of Marriage and Family Counselors, and a member of the American Counseling Association. Dr. Gray has authored eleven best selling books and he is an internationally recognized expert in the fields of communication and relationships. John Gray's unique focus is assisting men and women in understanding, respecting, and appreciating their differences. For more than thirty years he has conducted public and private seminars for thousands of participants. In his highly acclaimed books, audio tapes, and videos, as well as his seminars Dr. Gray entertains and inspires audiences with his practical insights and easy to use communication techniques that can be immediately applied to enrich relationships. John Gray is a popular speaker on The National Lecture Circuit and often appears on television and radio programs to discuss his work. He has made guest appearances on such shows as *Oprah, Good Morning America, The Today Show, Live With Regis, The View, Politically Incorrect, Larry King Live, The Roseanne Show, CNN and Company,* and many others. He has been profiled in *USA Today, Time Magazine, Forbes,* and numerous major newspapers across the United States. Dr. Gray welcome to *Conversations on Health and Wellness.*

Dr. John Gray (Gray)
Well, it's a real pleasure. Thank you.

Wright
You are the best selling relationship author of all time, but your latest book is about diet and exercise. Why the change in direction?

Gray
Well, it's actually not a change in direction it is expanding the core message that I have been delivering for the last thirty years, which is how to have better relationships. Whether they be an intimate relationship, or a romantic relationship, or a relationship with your children, trying to find a relationship, healing from a past relationship, and a relationship with our self. What I discovered in all of those relationships is how we exercise and what we put in our bodies. I found that the kind of exercise that we do, or the lack of exercise that we do, directly effects brain chemistry, and brain chemistry effects how we communicate. Also how we eat and our style of eating will dramatically affect how our brain functions. If you want to have affective communication in a relationship optimal brain function is the primary foundation. If I come into my marriage with my wife and I have no energy and I'm tired, she's not going to get what she's used to getting in the relationship. If she is feeling frustrated and over whelmed, or depressed there is no way I'm going to get the same kind of support that I'm used to getting. What I see happen to many couples over time is that men tend to lose that passion that they felt in the beginning for the relationship, and the interest in her tends to wane. He may love her, but that energy that they had in the beginning tends to dissipate. With women, that willingness to be flexible and open to change, optimism and appreciation that they felt in the beginning gradually gets numbed and turns into more of an occasional resentments towards their partner and an inability to appreciate and forgive their partner for their mistakes. These functions that are psychological functions I just said are directly related to brain function. And brain function is directly related to what kind of exercise we did that day and what we eat, what we had for breakfast particularly.

Wright

How does health issues such as diet and exercise help in understanding the opposite sex?

Gray

I'm going to turn it around on you. Understanding the opposite sex helps us to realize what's going on in our bodies. For example, one of the common things that men will experience and say not always directly to a women. I wouldn't recommend that, but when men are talking they'll often say things like "Gosh, she got so upset over nothing. She's making a big deal out of this. I can't understand why she's so bothered by this." And sometimes men say that directly to women. Which is a number one communication stopper. These kinds of messages sound condescending, and from a women's point of view they are. A man's brain functions differently than a woman's. It's only been in the last ten years that this has been verified by advanced technology that can actually scan the brain and measure blood flow in the brain during different emotional states. What they've found is that the limbic system of the brain, which is the emotional center, tends to be twice as big in women than in men. Eight times more blood will flow to the limbic system when a woman becomes upset about something. So naturally she is going to have a stronger emotional reaction. What men don't understand is that when she has a stronger emotional reaction it doesn't mean she's saying that the problem is bigger than he is saying it is.

Lets say the problem is you lost ten cents. A woman is going to have eight times more blood flowing to the brain if she lost ten cents than a man would. You see these kind of differences between men and women and then you start finding that there's actual hormonal differences in our bodies and brains and actual brain differences that give rise to different types of emotional and mental reactions to things. When we see that, then we look at how our diet and exercise effect brain function. If you want better relationships you need to understand the way that our brains and bodies function, feed and nurture the body because that's the basis of our skills in relating. When we talk about health and wellness if you're not feeling happy, if you're not feeling positive in your life much of the time, your body just can not sustain health. Likewise, if you're not taking care of your health and your health is going down hill it's very hard to feel fully alive and happy and fulfilled. It's all directly interrelated. If a person's motivation is to have a better relationship, they need to take particular care of their health and their optimal brain functioning. If somebody is only caring about their health they can enormously improve their health by improving their relationships. There are studies that show that by helping couples improve their communication skills it directly affected and improved optimal brain functioning. It's all directly related.

Wright

You have stated and I quote, "The magic key to health, happiness, and romance is waiting for you in your local health food store." What do you mean?

Gray

Well, I love that statement in the book. If you go into your health food store or any vitamin shop there are so many products. There are so many things waiting for you to try. Some of them may have benefits for people, but they are not all directly relevant to every person walking in. So you might say, "What do I start with?" Some things work and some things don't work. Why don't they? There's a lot of confusion. What I've done is develop a plan to shown people the basic ingredients for producing optimal brain chemistry. I list out what those ingredients are. Go into your health food store and put them all together in a morning shake because it's in the morning for breakfast that the brain is primarily producing optimal brain chemistry, which will set the direction for the rest of the day. If you don't start the day out in a clear space it's hard to regain it. Even for myself I always start out with a shake. Just put the ingredients in a shake and it taste really good. It's got your protein in it, it's got essential fatty acids in it, it's got enzymes in it, it's got trace minerals in it, it's got healthy carbohydrates in it, it's got your basic vitamins, particularly your B vitamins that are required to produce dopamine and serotonin in the brain. You get all of these basic ingredients in the right balance to each other and in good quality. Those are your three things you want quality, quantity, and balance. Particularly when you look at men and women, men need more protein, and women need more fat. If women have too much protein that will inhibit the production of serotonin, which produces feelings of well being. If men have too much fat in theirs that will prohibit the production of dopamine and they will tend to feel lethargic so we need to find the right balance. I've worked out a simple formula for people. They can make that morning shake and immediately they are on the road to experiencing optimal brain function.

Wright

I read, and you stated, that dopamine deficiency in men can cause emotional withdraw, romantic withdraw, excessive or deficiency in energy, addictive behavior, and even infidelity. So how do men reverse these effects?

Gray

Well it's very simple. This program is designed to start helping the brain produce the chemicals it needs to produce. When men are getting enough protein in the morning with the enzymes to break down those proteins, and the trace minerals to activate the enzymes, and the omega three essential fatty acids to convert those amino acids into dopamine, your brain starts producing normal amounts of dopamine.

When we are low in dopamine we have an addictive tendency. Almost all addictions are associated with dopamine levels in the brain. Dopamine gives us a since of pleasure and energy. I mentioned before that low serotonin takes away our sense of peacefulness, and optimism, and relaxation, and creates food cravings for food, called emotional eating. Low dopamine tends to make us tried. We have low energy, so we then have food cravings for sugar, energy, or anything that will produce dopamine. Beer and alcohol for some people immediately convert into dopamine.

For some people when you have low dopamine, you look for opportunities or more intense experiences in order to stimulate production of dopamine. The same thing is true of men walking around with low dopamine if they meet a new woman. New and different woman stimulates dopamine, but once you get to know her then she's not new and different anymore. So it doesn't stimulate the dopamine anymore. If you are low in dopamine, at that point you lose interest in her. If you're not low in dopamine you never lose interest. You're able to sustain that interest for a lifetime. So what happens in passionate relationships is that you generally have about three years of free dopamine. In the beginning she's new and different and everything's new and different. Also, challenges are one thing that stimulates dopamine too. So, the relationship's a challenge and she's new and different, and you tend to get a lot of rewards in the beginning. These are things that stimulate dopamine. But after about three years routine sets in and then dopamine doesn't get produced in a situation of routine. So the same guy who has low dopamine has low interest in the relationship. It doesn't mean he doesn't love his wife. He can love her completely. Love is another hormone than dopamine. But he goes to work and suddenly he comes alive and he's got energy, he's got motivation, he's got clarity, he's got interest, and he comes home and he's kind of just interested in watching TV and being passive. What is that? Well that is just a symptom of low dopamine, and generally there are three factors that cause that. One is the style of communication between him and his wife. This can immediately lower dopamine levels. Two the kind of exercise or lack of exercise he did that day can lower dopamine levels. And three what he eats for breakfast can raise or lower dopamine levels.

People are always saying, "exercise, exercise." I'm not the person who says, "exercise, exercise" I'm saying do the right kind of exercise. If a man does too much exercise that will lower his dopamine levels. Dopamine is produced by amino acids and those very same amino acids are also used by the body to restore muscle mass. So if you're breaking down muscles by lifting weights everyday than you are not going to have enough amino acids available to produce dopamine in the brain.

Cocaine produces dopamine as well. Then once you are done the dopamine levels drop way down and you lose interest. So these things can all be corrected, like with weightlifting, I do weightlifting myself. I only do it once a week for twenty minutes. I also know that for the next twenty-four hours I won't be able to function with full brain capacity, but that's okay I like to keep my muscle mass, and it's good to work out. There is even research today that shows that just working out once a week by fully exhausting your seven or eight muscle groups just in two to three minutes each, simple, easy, slow movements, you actually build muscle more affectively than if you were working out three times a day.

Wright

You know one person that read your book and reviewed it got great results from it. That same person is trying your formula on their son who has had severe allergies and asthma. Have any of your readers had success with asthma or allergies?

Gray

I get antidotal reports of it all the time. I think that my program is not designed to cure allergies or asthma, however, it is designed to assist people in getting the nutrients they need for balanced brain chemicals. When you have balanced brain chemicals it tends to be easier to eat a balanced diet, which doesn't include a lot of refined carbohydrates. I know for a fact, or at least in my life, if you eat a lot of sugary products it will really make allergies and asthma much, much worse. If you are getting the nutrients that your body needs, those health symptoms tend to become minimized. I'm not claiming that this program cures anything, but I know I hear all of these reports of people that say these conditions are helped or cleared up very quickly.

The body can be healthier when the brain is functioning the way it is designed to function. The brain is really the executive system of the whole body. When the brain's not working the body just shuts down to a certain extent. We need to have that optimal brain function. We need to eat healthier foods. We need to make sure we move our bodies enough. We need to make sure we are getting enough oxygen to our body. You can just see that the normal sedentary life style of Americans. They don't get what they are needing, so naturally their body, particularly over forty, starts degenerating.

Even now with our children breathing in all of the pollutants, all the types of food colorings, food additives, toxins that we have, the massive amounts of food, and that sugar issue, we eat so much of it the body becomes allergic to it. Sugar is in everything. So that activates allergies quite a bit. The program I suggested is not one of telling your kids they can never eat sugar again, but that of coming back to a very moderate type of on "special occasions" they can have ice cream, cake or cookies, as opposed to everyday. Our kids have these food cravings, and the food cravings can be corrected with this program. It helps people feel satisfied with what they have and tends to create a stronger desire for healthier food.

If you're a boy and you've got plenty of dopamine in your brain, you're not tired. When the kids are tired or bored they want the high intense soda drinks. When they get older they want their coffee, and all of these types of stimulants to give them energy. One of the things people tell me all of the time is they don't drink coffee anymore when they have this morning shake. It's not like they had to go off of coffee, they just don't want coffee. They don't need it. They don't feel that need because what coffee will do is give you a burst of dopamine, but then it's gone. See these things that raise your blood sugar, they stimulate your body and you will get energy from that, but it doesn't last. The program that I am suggesting will balance your hormones as opposed to throwing them out of balance.

Wright

You have reported that if men and women eat the same thing there will likely be fights and disappointments that send them into orbit, just as when men and women tried to communicate in love making without taking into consideration male and female differences. Can you explain what you mean?

Gray

What I mean there is that we need to have a communication style that includes our partner's different style. You know I have my own way of communicating, but I need to realize that when she's talking that she speaks another language. I can't make her language wrong, and I'm not saying my language is better than hers, I'm trying to interpret the best I can what she's saying and vice versa. Understanding our differences in relationships makes a huge difference. Now I take that to another level, which is understanding our different nutritional needs. There are certain vulnerabilities that women have today when it comes to food. One of the big ones is not getting enough fat and eating to much protein. I've interviewed lots of women when I give my talks in different cities, and I sign hundreds of books wherever I go of people reading the book and hearing my talk. They're all asking me questions about their diet, and about their relationships and so forth.

I remember doing one in Tennessee. The first eight women camp up to say that they had been making some good progress on the Adkins diet, but had some questions how this fit in with that or something. In Adkins they are following a high protein diet low carbohydrates. I would say, "What's your mood? How do you feel on this diet?" They would say, "Well okay, but you know I also take Prozac, Zoloft, or something similar. I'd say, "Well when did you start that?" Every single one of these women had started about a couple of weeks to a couple of months after doing the Adkins diet. The reason I bring this up is I said, "Do you think there's any link to what you are eating and your depression?" It was the first time they had considered that. It's so irresponsible for a doctor even to prescribe a Prozac or a Zoloft without asking a person, "What do you eat for breakfast? What is the amount of protein that you are eating in you diet?" What these women learned is that if you eat too much protein it will cause depression. You may lose weight because you're getting all of these calories of protein and the fat that goes with it, so you are getting satisfied with that. You are not putting on weight because you're not eating any carbohydrates. You can't knock carbohydrates out of your diet. Carbohydrates, rice, grains and pasta—that's your choice. But you've got to eat vegetables, and that's carbohydrates. This is the fuel for the brain. The brain can only burn sugar. This is why I teach the fat burning exercises. It's to train the muscles how to burn fat again so that the sugar is left for the brain because the brain needs lots of sugar to burn. It can't burn fat, but the kind of stressful lives we live particularly the kind of exercise we do or lack of exercise tends to cause us to burn sugar all of the time instead of burning fat. So when the body muscles are burning fat there is plenty of sugar in the brain, and that sugar comes ideally from complex carbohydrates instead of the refined sugars.

On the other hand, when women eat excess protein the blood is filled with all the amino acids. The amino acids break down the protein. The smallest of these amino acids is something called tryptophan. Tryptophan is what converts into serotonin, and because it is the smallest of the amino acids it is the last to get into the brain. There is what is called the blood brain barrier and only a certain amount of amino acids can get into the brain. The bigger ones go in first and they block the little ones. So if you have a lot of proteins for a woman she's going to experience less tryptophan getting into her brain to produce serotonin.

Now men don't have this problem because they have a greater muscle mass. So when they eat a lot of protein the muscle mass absorbs many of those long chain proteins so that the short chain tryptophan can easily get into the brain. But research shows this tends to synthesize serotonin, which comes from tryptophan, twice as fast as women. Men tend to store twice as much tryptophan in their brains, which means we don't use it up as fast. Again, as we talked about earlier in the interview, women have a bigger emotional center in the brain when it becomes excited, which means more blood flow to the brain. The brain has to then produce more serotonin to relax the emotions. So women use up their serotonin much faster than men, and they also have more difficulty producing the serotonin, particularly with the average American diet which is so high protein.

So women particularly need balance, not that you can ever achieve perfect balance unless you are making it in your morning shake. But as a rough guide, if you think in terms of calories, about half of your calories need to be complex carbohydrates or carbohydrates for women, about twenty percent ideally protein, and about thirty percent ideally good fat. For men, about thirty percent protein and twenty percent good fat. This is not a hard and fast rule, it's a generally guide line. Just a little more protein for men and a little less fat for men, and a little more fat for women and a little less protein is the secret to making sure you are getting the right balance of nutrients.

But it's not just that, it is other factors you need to make sure you are getting enough B vitamins and trace minerals. You need to make sure that you have the enzymes to digest the protein, and you need to make sure that every morning you eat a complete protein. So when you get all of those things together you do have the formula for optimal brain functioning. You see all kind of benefits in adults.

As you mentioned, people write in and they tell me children are benefiting so much from this. Particularly the kids with the A.D.D. symptoms. In boys with the A.D.D. symptoms, the results are very dramatic because you see it right away. All of these low dopamine symptoms I talked about with men have low energy and needing risk, challenge, danger, new and different to stimulate the dopamine. The symptom of low dopamine in kids is what we now commonly call A.D.D. It's attention deficit disorder or attention deficit hyperactive disorder, which basically means you put a child in a classroom and they get bored, restless, and they don't think clearly anymore. If you take that same child and you put him in front of a video game and the brain functions perfectly or ideally, that is because the video game has the challenge, the danger, has the risk, has the new and different, has the rewards and that stimulates the dopamine. But a healthy child shouldn't need that kind of stimulation to experience interest and pleasure.

For men, when they have the low dopamine it tends to be more like "I don't have the energy to get things done," or "I don't have enough stimulation." or "I'm bored with this I need more stimulation." So the symptoms are very, very different once you understand how men and women's brains are different, how are fat to muscle mass differential is different these things all have huge impact on our psychology and our state of health, and our sense of well-being particularly does romance thrive. The huge aspect of living a long healthy life is making sure that you have passion. If you don't have that passion, and you don't have optimism and well-being (passion coming from dopamine and well-being and optimism coming from serotonin) your brain's just not functioning in a manner that will allow your body to stay healthy.

Wright

Well what a great conversation. This was all very interesting. I wish that we had all day, but I know you've got a thousand things to do. I really do appreciate the time you've taken with me today and I've learned a lot. Dr. Gray, thank you so much for being with us.

Gray

A real pleasure for my part, too.

About The Author

John Gray, Ph.D., is recognized internationally as a leader in the field of relationships and personal growth. For over twenty years he has conducted public and private seminars to enrich the quality of relationships and improve communications. His unique focus is assisting men and women in respecting and accepting their differences.

Dr. John Gray

www.marsvenus.com

Chapter 3

DAVID M. JACOBSON, MSW

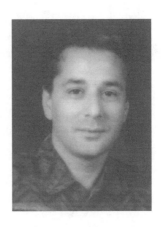

THE INTERVIEW

David E. Wright (Wright)

Today we are talking to David Jacobson. David was diagnosed with a severe form of arthritis at age 22. He attributes conquering his illness and going from barely being able to walk to accomplishing a 50-mile unicycle ride to his humor and positive lifestyle. Mr. Jacobson has a diverse background as a master's level social worker, former athlete, former top sales director and trainer, and former college of medicine and graduate school instructor. David's greatest accomplishment was being chosen one of only 50 national heroes by the Arthritis Foundation out of thousands of nominations. The National Hero Overcoming Arthritis Award is presented for outstanding courage and inspiration in meeting the challenges of arthritis. David has won numerous awards in the categories of Inspiration, Motivation, and Poetry. David has been presented with a joy mask from the Korean Broadcasting System for his contribution and participation in their exceptional documentary series on health and stress. As a recognized leader in the field of humor and health, David has been interviewed by news media of all forms in both the United States and internationally. David Jacobson, welcome to *Conversations on Health and Wellness*!

David Jacobson (Jacobson)
Thank you.

Wright
David, what are some of the benefits of using humor for health?

Jacobson
Oh, well there's a lot of benefits. There's physiological benefits, psychological, social, spiritual, economic all related to health. Physiologically, we're all aware of the stress response. The fight or flight syndrome. We've all felt it. Your heart starts to race. Your blood pressure goes up. Stomach acids increase. The mouth goes dry. Adrenaline amounts rise to give the body more fuel and energy. Your ability to digest food decreases so that more blood can flow to muscles. Muscle tension increases. Perspiration increases to cool the body. The spleen releases stored blood cells and cortisol, a blood clotting agent; and Lactic acid rushes to the muscles for added strength. The liver releases glucose for energy. Your breathing becomes shallower, your personality becomes shallower, your chances of winning the lottery decreases... it's just a terrible mess all around! If stress continues to go unchecked for any period of time, eventually your resistance to disease and infections will be lowered and your health will be in jeopardy and I'm not talking Alex Trebek.

There are a lot of negative effects from that stress. When that high level of stress occurs and your heart rate's increased and your muscles become tense, adrenalin flows through the blood, there's something we need to do to counteract that so that we aren't under such heavy stress. There's many ways to do that. Some people have used meditation to induce a relaxation response, but I've found that laughter is the greatest antidote. There are no side effects and it's very good for you. (Well there might be one side effect if you laugh too hard, but rubber panties will solve that one.) Think about when you have a hearty laugh, and you're just cracking up and going, ah ha uhh, taking those deep breaths when you're laughing like that and oxygenating your blood. Your blood pressure initially shoots up during your laughter, but afterwards decreases below normal. Research shows that people that laugh hearty on a regular basis have lower standing blood pressures than the average population. It also decreases your muscle tension. There's evidence that laughter stimulates the production of catecholamines, the alertness hormones, and laughter may even cause the release of endorphins which are natural pain killers. This could improve your ability to tolerate pain. You've heard of the runners high. There's certain things that induce this altered state and laughter is one of them, and much less strenuous than running a marathon.

Wright

What are some of the psychological benefits?

Jacobson

Well, psychologically, when you have an illness like arthritis or any type of disease, you're going to have losses associated with that. With my arthritis, I suffered a lot of losses. I lost my favorite hobbies. You've mentioned the athletic part of me. I was in Judo and bicycling, mountain climbing, cliff diving, running, jogging—all of those physical activities. I lost my role as an athlete. I couldn't do any of those things any more. I lost a pain-free body. I lost that strong athletic build and even the ability to just sleep straight through the night. I had a high level of energy before the illness. I didn't afterwards. I lost my self-confidence and self-esteem that were tied to that physical body. So I lost that joyful personality, that positive outlook on life when I was diagnosed. I lost my wallet, but that's a different story. I won't get into that. But basically psychologically humor can be used to replace those losses that you feel when you're having an illness. One way to replace those losses is to use your mind or to change the way you think about the situation. So I found some ways to replace those losses.

An example is my first week of work—you mentioned me being a social worker, I was the emergency room social worker at the University Medical Center here in Tucson. My first week of work was the holiday week of Christmas. There were a lot of traumas. There were motor vehicle accidents, gunshot wounds, and death in the ER. It was just a horrible week, and we had our first meeting of all the social workers. My boss, the manager there, Danny Blake, asked me, "So, David, how did your first week of work go?" And words couldn't describe that week, so I just collapsed on the floor. Outwardly, people were chuckling a little bit and they kind of got the joke that describes a little better than saying anything. Later people came up to Danny and said, "Gee, who'd you hire this time?" But they actually appreciated that. I had people pat me on the back and say, "Hey, thanks for making the usual boring meeting a little lighter this time." So I got some self-confidence and self-esteem from that that I used to get from physical activities I could now get through my sense of humor. So I was able to replace the losses by using the humor. There is a powerful relationship between how you perceive what is happening to you (the threat) and what is going on biochemically in your body. Using humor to confront whatever the perceived threat is will ease tension and provide you with the ability to see things from a new perspective.

With every event or situation, psychologically, we know it's not the event that causes the stress, it's how we perceive it. So if you can use humor to change the way you perceive a situation, you're going to have a psychological benefit from doing that. By sustaining a more positive mood, and reducing the amount of time spent in a state of anger, anxiety or depression, you can play an active role in mobilizing your body's own health and healing forces. Your emotional state begins working for you, rather than against.

Wright

I see you spoke about spirituality. How is humor related to spirituality?

Jacobson

Well, for me, I have a hard time separating my humor from my spirituality. They are two sides of the same coin because I've seen that my own personal belief system encompasses humor as part of my purpose for being here. I feel that's part of my purpose on this planet is to use my humorous side to inspire others. That in turn fuels my passion and drive to continue spreading the message about humors positive qualities. I've always gone by that cosmic joke of the universe philosophy. It's kind of been a theme of my life where there's a spirit of laughter. We've heard of the spirit of the dance, the team spirit, the spirit of alcohol. Well, there's a spirit of laughter also, and it's universal. It's something that all humans do. So even if you don't speak the same language, people can go into a theater and watch Charlie Chaplin's slap stick comedy, and laugh. So what it does is it decreases prejudice and reveals how much closer all of us as human beings are to each other.

Through the spirit of laughter we are connected to each other. Our sense of humor helps to reveal that inner connection we have with each other and those that are sensitive to it can actually feel that connection when sharing joy with others.

Wright

I remember the universal joke years ago when the "God is dead" theory came about, and someone said, "If he is dead, then he must have laughed himself to death watching us."

Jacobson

Hey we are pretty silly when you think about it. That message about not taking life too seriously; I don't take myself seriously. I might take the things I do serious, if it's a profession or a situation or something, I can take that seriously, but I don't have to take what I do seriously. There's some exercises that are I like to call humor building exercises that people can do to strengthen their sense of humor and that kind of humorous spiritual philosophy.

Wright

What are some of the humor strategies and techniques people can use to improve their health?

Jacobson

Well, the first one isn't really a strategy. It's a mindset, and this is attributed to C. W. Metcalf, who co-authored a book with Roma Felible called, *Lighten Up: Survival Skills for People Under Pressure.* One point he makes is that the first thing we as humans have to do is overcome our fear of foolishness. Most of us are afraid of embarrassment and what we will look like in public. There's a lot of cultural and societal rules about laughter. Can you just laugh when you're sitting in a doctor's office or walking down the street? There's a lot of times where people would be embarrassed if they're laughing in public even. So the first thing we must do is just overcome that fear.

Wright

I'm reminded of one of the funniest scenes on television ever recorded that won all kinds of awards. They play it at least once a year, it was when Mary Tyler Moore laughed at a funeral of the clown that died.

Jacobson

Yes, I remember that.

Wright

We've all been there.

Jacobson

Yeah! That's a great example. It's really true. There's times when it is and it isn't okay to laugh in public too, but the more comfortable we are with our laughter, the healthier we'll be. People have had heart attacks working themselves up into a frenzy by negative, fearful or angry thoughts. Here is an example of a strategy I developed as a result of my arthritis. I have to walk with a limp sometimes. My first step in becoming healthy again was literally a humorous one and that was the silly walk. I don't know if you've seen Monty Python's department of silly walks?

Wright

Yes I have.

Jacobson

That's one example of it. But basically, I figured if I have to walk slowly and with a limp, I might as well have fun doing it. So I exaggerated my walk to the point of being ridiculous. When I was first diagnosed with severe arthritis it took weeks to become strong enough to get in a wheelchair and return to the States from Israel where I had gotten sick. I was 22 and just beginning to walk again. My mother was like an Edith Bunker type mom. She did everything. When the phone would ring, "Oh, don't get up David, I'll get it." She ran around doing the laundry and cooking. What I really needed at that point was to take an independent step. So what I did was I wanted to beat her to the phone. I had a plan. So when the phone rang and she said, "Oh, don't get up, I'll get it," I kind of dragged myself like Igor on the knuckles of my right hand touching the floor, I hobbled to the phone. She was so busy laughing, I beat her to it. That was kind of the realization to me. I've got this painful body, but that doesn't mean I can't have fun living in it. Another strategy that's related to this is getting into the witness state. Getting out of yourself so you can see it from a different perspective, from a fresh and better way, a better perspective. My feeling joyful at watching my mother laugh for the first time since I returned home in such an unhealthy state, helped me see things from a new perspective.

Wright

Did you say the "witness" state?

Jacobson

Yes, the witness state. If you've ever seen *Fiddler on the Roof*, they show Tevya going into the witness state. Whenever he's got to make a decision, everything would freeze, and then he'd say, "Hum, let's look at this side of it, and let's look at that side of it." So I use that as my example. If I can get out of this situation because when you are emotionally caught up in it, there's not a lot of objective judgment there. You can't do much with it, but if you can separate yourself from your emotions you can be more objective. That's actually another strategy, becoming an actor or becoming your favorite comedian. So I would become Dustin Hoffman and be the actor in the scene. By that, an example is let's say my wife and I are quarreling, and she's angry. I'm angry. Well, she might say something in anger, and I'll say "Freeze! Cut!" I'll say, "That was perfect. You would have won an Academy Award with that! Do that again." It's very hard to repeat because you are now aware of trying to act.

Wright

Right.

Jacobson

This helps you to not be emotionally involved in the anger. You are more aware of watching yourself and you're aware of what you're doing. That's pretty helpful.

Wright

You spoke a moment ago of inappropriate, what makes humor appropriate or inappropriate?

Jacobson

The basic rule for appropriate humor is anything that's inclusive is appropriate if it brings people together. A healthy humor builds people up. It comes from a place of caring or empathy. It encourages a positive atmosphere. These are appropriate types of humor. So it's kind of common sense, but a lot of people don't have common sense unfortunately. Usually inappropriate humor is done out of ignorance. It's not usually done to purposely be mean, but inappropriate humor is more the exclusive humor. It divides people or it reinforces stereotypes. It's not healthy. It's based on ignorance or insensitivity.

Wright

I remember, I don't do it anymore, but I remember hearing many years ago what I thought was funny. This friend of mine walked up to me and said, "You know, David, boy that's a great looking tie. Did you buy it new?" I laughed, but then I used it several times after that and I figured out this is inappropriate. They're not laughing. They think I'm serious here.

Jacobson

It's hard. Sometimes one good thing to base it on is how well you know the person. Like I'm sure, David, the people that are your friends or relatives that know you know exactly what you mean and where you are coming from.

Wright

Right.

Jacobson

The people that don't know you as well can take things wrong.

Wright

Absolutely. How do you deal with inappropriate humor?

Jacobson

Well, I think dealing with it depends on your personality style, the type of mood you're in at the time, just a lot of different factors. One way is to just simply choose not to laugh. You know someone tells an inappropriate joke, they'll get the message that you don't find it funny if you give them a serious look instead of a laugh. You can be a little more assertive and say, "You know, I don't find that kind of humor funny. I don't think it's funny." They probably won't use that around you again. If you want room to, like I mentioned, some people aren't aware that they are doing that, give them a chance to save face by saying something like, "Well, I'm sure you're not aware of how mean spirited that joke is or how that makes you sound. You probably wouldn't use it if you realized that." You can use it as an educational thing too. One way I've used it to educate others is if it is a stereotypical joke, you know racist, sexist, religious, I'll say, "Okay tell that joke again but use your own group in the example." All of a sudden they realize well then it's not funny and an "aha" goes off. I had to educate them.

Wright

How did poetry relate to humor in your healing process?

Jacobson

Poetry can be very therapeutic. The poetry I write is funny poetry basically. When I've had a massive flare-up and I'm stuck in bed for a couple of weeks or something like that, I had to have my vent out and the poetry was one. I wrote a poem that is an example of that. It's kind of my whole philosophy in a poem called *A Place for Pain*. It goes like this:

> *I open the door, pain walks in filling my home with darkness and discontent.*
> *I open the door, love walks in replenishing the bed-room.*
> *I open the door, faith walks in illuminating my living room.*
> *I open the door, hope walks in filling the kitchen with wonderful smells.*
> *I open the door, joy walks in. I explain that she has the wrong address.*
> *She should be next door. She comes in anyway. Joy, like pain, knows*
> *not of manners or proper protocol.*
> *I open the door, humor walks in. It fills the empty spaces.*
> *Pain is still here but it has little room.*

So that was my way of encompassing all of the positive aspects of our life. We need hope. For some people, faith is more important than the humor or joy, whichever, love. You know some people look for their family. That's their drive to keep going, and that's my way of kind of summing that up.

Wright

It's a great poem.

Jacobson

Thank you.

Wright

How do you use humor to take the next step from just overcoming and managing your health to actually thriving?

Jacobson

Well, again, I think that's different for everyone, but yet how I did it was I found that I tried to see what makes me different than most, and it wasn't any incredible will power or super human ability to tolerate pain. I've got average intelligence, my wife and mother might say I'm a little smarter than the average bear, but there's a lot of depressed intelligent people out there. There's a lot of depressed wealthy people or successful people out there. It comes from something else, and what it is, I think, is my daily thoughts are much different than most. You try to think of silly things every day. If you're out looking through those humor filtered glasses of seeing the absurdities of life in all of your interactions, if you can do that, you'd be so much healthier. It would be incredible. I think it's a strong boost to the immune system. I think I have not very much stress because I can do this. Those events we talked about that causes stress are much less stressful for me. There's much less stress in my life because I have a strategy of taking a negative situation and finding the positive within it. Whenever we're in a negative situation, we kind of "awfullize" it. Like that, "Oh, I'm having another flare-up so I'm going to be in pain and I'm going to be miserable and tortured, and this is going to happen, and that." If you can find the positive within the situation, sort of like my poetry, the last time I had a flare-up I wrote some pretty neat poems. So I can try to look at the positive and say, "Oh, look! I'm going to get a little break. I'm going to get to rest now, and I'm going to be able to write" or whatever the situation is.

Wright

How can humor be used by those with chronic illnesses to educate others regarding disability?

Jacobson

Well, I think that's okay to educate people that are inquisitive, or even nosy, about what's wrong with someone who is disabled. Those situations come up quite often in my handicap parking or places like that. What I do is I try to point out that arthritis is an invisible disease and you can't always see the pain, and I use the parking lot situation sometimes to educate depending on my mood, if I'm in that mood. It's important to realize that I don't really owe someone an explanation, but on good days you can really use it as an educational point to make someone more aware about disabilities. An example is a friend of mine who has a child with arthritis. He was pushing his child in a wheelchair and someone said, "Gee, I didn't know kids can get arthritis." It was probably the 100 thousandth time he'd heard that statement. So he will respond seriously and say, "Oh yes, and the fact that we live on a power line tree house probably doesn't help either." If he gets that reaction, David, that you just gave, if he gets a laugh, he goes on to educate them and say, "Yeah," and then he gives them actual facts about it. Some people just give him a blank look, the ones that don't get it, and then he's done because they're not, in his mind, worth explaining to because they really don't get it. But if someone's got a sense of humor, and they can laugh at that, then he'll take the time to educate them. He uses the humor to be the opening point for the education.

Wright
By the way, how is your health now?

Jacobson
Oh, it's really good, thanks. I'm off all the strong medications I used to be on and I'm doing pretty good.

Wright
So you're thriving instead of surviving.

Jacobson
Exactly. Yeah, I would say I'm thriving right now.

Wright
That's great. What resources are available to learn more about humor and health?

Jacobson
Well, the first one that comes to mind is related to the last question. There's a book by John Callahan called *Don't Worry, He Won't Get Far on Foot.*

Wright
Don't worry?

Jacobson
He's a quadriplegic, if anyone doesn't know that. So on his book cover is this wheelchair turned over, this drag mark in the sand, and

two police looking over the wheelchair saying, "Don't worry he won't get far on foot."

Wright

That's funny.

Jacobson

Yeah, so that cover kind of sums up his philosophy. He describes his adjustment to becoming quadriplegic in a really humorous way. At the end of the book, he does just what you asked me in the last question. He uses his cartooning abilities to educate others about disability, teaching them about disability and things like that are in the book. So that's a good resource. There are other good books. You mentioned the Mary Tyler Moore scene. That reminded me of the Steve Allen scene a long time ago when he cracked up on his show and couldn't stop laughing. He wrote a book, *How to Be Funny*, and a lot of people can use a book like that to learn some more techniques about how to be funnier. *The Healing Power of Humor* by Allen Klein is also an excellent book on the subject of humor and health. ... and of course, you know the classics are Norman Cousins' books, *Anatomy of an Illness* and *Head First*.

Wright

Yeah, my wife is a cancer survivor and I think the Norman Cousin book kept her alive.

Jacobson

Really?

Wright

Yeah.

Jacobson

Wow!

Wright

As a matter of fact they were required reading at the rehabilitation that she took. Norman is just great.

Jacobson

I agree. It's really true and what he said in the book was true for me. When I have a flare-up, if I could crack up for ten minutes straight, I could get a couple of hours of pain-free sleep. That was better than the narcotics could do. So yeah, it's really true what he says. There's more books on actual humor skills like Gene Perret. He's written some books. *Comedy Writing Step by Step* is one of his books. He's got a lot of comedy books on just the skills and techniques. Anyone can develop their sense of humor. It goes back to the human spirituality. We all have it. We all have a sense of humor. Some of us have developed it more than others.

Wright

Gene wrote for Bob Hope for many, many, many years.

Jacobson

Yes, he did. Yeah, he was his writer, and an excellent one too. Yeah. Any books by your favorite comedians are great books to read because it gives you a better chance to see the world through their eyes, and then you'll see the world more humorously if you do that. We all have different tastes in humor like we do in food and any other subject. So you have to find what works for you.

Wright

You talked about spirituality. Down through the years throughout your life, as you have made your decisions, has faith played an important role in your life?

Jacobson

I think so, yeah. I think that getting the arthritis, or any illness will have an effect on your personality. But significant parts of you don't go away. They just manifest in a different way. The fate was getting diagnosed with severe arthritis at a young age. The benefit of it, because there's always benefits when there's tragic parts, is that I really developed my sense of humor and I really developed an outlook on life that I know will help me survive through any kind of tragedy. So yeah, I think that certain things are meant to be so that we develop stronger as humans. Then we can be placed in a position to help others from what we have learned. That applies to everyone. We all have teachings that others are in need of.

Wright

I'm going to have to go get that book, *He Won't Get Far on Foot* just to see the front cover. That might be one of the funniest things I've heard in a few weeks.

Jacobson

Yes. There's a few different front covers he's done on it, but that's the funny one. It's a good book.

Wright

What a great conversation and what an enlightening conversation. I really appreciate, David, the time you've taken out of your day to talk to us and give us all this information laced with a lot of humor, I might add.

Jacobson

Thanks, I really enjoyed it. Thank you.

Wright

Today we have been talking to David Jacobson who was diagnosed with a severe form of arthritis at 22, but as we have found today, there are probably several reasons he's won all of these awards and citations. We find him now, under my definition, thriving instead of just surviving. Thank you so much, David, for being with us on *Conversations on Health and Wellness*!

Jacobson

You're welcome.

About The Author

David M. Jacobson, MSW has been a healthcare professional for twenty years and is a professional speaker who specializes in humor and health. He is married and has four children. Of all his honors and awards the Wayne Washburn Award says it best: "We all need someone or something to inspire us to bring out our best. You are that someone."

David M. Jacobson, MSW
President: Humor Horizons
4745 S. Paseo Melodioso
Tucson, Arizona 85730
Phone: 520-370-2203
Email: dj@humorhorizons.com
www.humorhorizons.com

Chapter 4

BARBARA THOMPSON

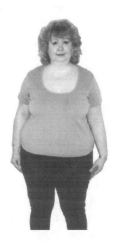 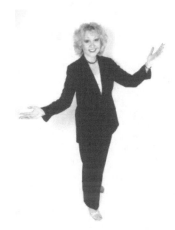

THE INTERVIEW

David E. Wright (Wright)

Today we are talking to Barbara Thompson, a recognized expert on obesity and weight loss surgery. Barbara is known as the pioneer in patient education. Her best selling book, *Weight Loss Surgery, Finding the Thin Person Hiding Inside You* has been dubbed the "unofficial bible of bypass patients" by the *Philadelphia Inquirer*.

Barbara Thompson battled a weight problem from the day she was born, only to diet her way to morbid obesity. When her weight reached 264 pounds, and a herniated disk in her back was causing her to face disability, she knew she was in trouble. She decided to have the life-altering gastric bypass surgery in January 2000.

Barbara is sought after nationally as a speaker and motivator. Through her speaking, Barbara brings hope to the dangerously obese, and stresses the right for personal dignity at any weight. Barbara, welcome to *Conversations on Health and Wellness.*

Barbara Thompson (Thompson)

Thank you very much, David.

Wright

You know, looking at your before and after pictures on the cover of your book, *Weight Loss Surgery: Finding the Thin Person Hiding Inside You*, it's obvious that the change in the way you look is drastic to say the least. How much weight did you lose and over what period of time?

Thompson

My highest weight was 264 pounds. I have lost 125 pounds since having weight loss surgery in January of 2000. Actually the weight loss is not what is so significant in my life. I've always been able to lose weight. What I've never been able to do, until now, is maintain that weight loss. I have kept that weight off in the years since my surgery. And to address the second part of that question, the weight loss was fairly dramatic. I lost that weight over a period of 11 months. So, I went from being morbidly obese to being of normal weight in less than a year. Adjusting to all of the changes that go along with that was significant. I had a difficult adjustment losing that amount of weight so rapidly. For instance, it's very disconcerting to be walking past a plate glass window, catch your reflection, and not recognize yourself. Then there's the matter of clothes. You lose your comfort clothes—those outfits that we put on and feel so comfortable and safe in. They literally start to fall off. It's like shedding a skin and leaving it behind. The whole idea of your own personal space changes and it takes a long time for your perceived image of yourself to catch up with the changes in your body. You see yourself as being much larger than you are for a long time afterwards. When my husband and I took a Caribbean vacation this past winter, I went down a water slide for the first time since my surgery. My first thought as I approached the slide was the fear I would get stuck. I've been of normal weight for almost four years, yet I was still afraid I would get stuck.

Wright

You know, as I read your book I felt a little strange and embarrassed every time you referred to your morbid obesity. I'd have a hard time referring to anyone as obese. What effect did your weight have on your self-image?

Thompson

Morbid obesity, or obesity for that matter, is a diagnosis, not a value judgment. The diagnosis is based upon a calculation of your height in relationship to your weight. This calculation is called your Body Mass Index or BMI. There are many Body Mass Index calculators that can be found on the internet. However, to determine your own Body Mass Index, multiple your weight in pounds by 704.5., divide by your height in inches, and divide again by your height in inches. A BMI between 18.5 and 24.9 is considered normal. A BMI between 25 and 29.9 is overweight. A BMI of 30 to 39.9 is obese. And 40 and above is morbidly obese. That means a woman who is 5' 6" tall and weighs 186 pounds is obese. A man who is 6' tall and weighs 221 pounds is obese.

There's so much shame connected to the subject of obesity. One of the seven deadly sins is gluttony. We look at people who are very much overweight and we make a value judgment about them. We view them as being weak and lazy, as having no control and not caring about how they look when just the opposite is true. Virtually every obese person that you see has struggled with his or her weight. It's just that they've lost the battle. And when you consider that 60 percent of the population in this country is overweight and that obesity is increasing so rapidly, those very people who are looking at the obese in such a disdainful way are probably headed to obesity themselves.

But I know exactly how you feel about the term "obese." Before my current marriage, I was married to a man who died during a hospital stay from a pulmonary embolism. There was an autopsy; and in reading the autopsy report, he was referred to as an "obese male." I was insulted. I argued that he was a bit overweight, but was certainly not obese. And I was upset, because I felt that he was being judged as obese. But clinically, according to his BMI, he was in fact obese. But the label upset me. And of course, I remember the first time that I was told that I was morbidly obese. I am just over 5' 6." Weighing 264 pounds, my BMI was 42. A Body Mass Index of 40 or above is morbidly obese. After I heard that, I was shocked that I had gotten so out of control that I was morbidly obese. Morbid obesity implied to me that my weight could kill me; and I was correct. Left unchecked, my morbid obesity could have eventually killed me.

Wright

During the 20 years that you have said that you were overweight, did you ever feel that you were a lesser human being? For example, did you feel you were not hired for a job or you missed other opportunities because of your weight?

Thompson

Obesity is the last opportunity for the insensitive and the uninformed to exercise blatant discrimination. It's fertile ground. There are many comedians who make their living laughing at obese people. My weight did affect me professionally, but it was the insensitive comments that people would make that were worse. One day I heard my daughter teased because her mother was fat. That was far more hurtful than any lost job opportunity.

Wright

As you talk to other people who have serious weight problems, what are the largest concerns in their lives?

Thompson

The largest concern is health. Obesity is at the root of a host of diseases and medical conditions. Those who are obese are 12 times more likely to die suddenly than those of normal weight. They're six times more likely to develop heart disease, 10 times more likely to develop diabetes and are at a much greater risk of developing cancer, respiratory problems, gall bladder problems, sleep apnea, and acid reflux. Their health is critical. We spend 75 billion dollars every year on weight related illnesses. Prior to my weight loss surgery, I had a herniated disc in my back. I was in tremendous pain; but you don't die from a herniated disc. But I felt like I was on a precipice looking down at all those health issues facing me. I wanted to do something about my weight and get it under control before those health issues got to me.

Another issue facing those who are morbidly obese is an absence of a good quality of life. A year and a half after I had my surgery, I went on a 22 mile bike ride. It was on one of those glorious summer days and I rode on a tree lined trail. It was wonderful. I was pedaling along like the Wicked Witch of the West. I was having a ball. It was so extraordinary that I was able to do that when 18 months earlier I was nearly disabled because my extra 125 pounds of weight put such painful pressure on the herniated disc in my back. But as extraordinary as that bike ride was, it was just as extraordinary the day I stood at the bottom of my stairs in my home and raced to the top and didn't think that I was going to die. I could actually breathe. That ordinary act was extraordinary to me. And I find the same kinds of feelings from the thousands of people that I meet as I travel around the country speaking about obesity and weight loss surgery. The absence of so many of the ordinary things of life, those things that normal-weighted people take for granted, are very precious to those who are morbidly obese.

I remember talking with a woman who had surgery and was losing weight rapidly. One day she looked down and realized that she had crossed her legs and started to cry over a simple, ordinary thing like that. There are so many things lacking from their lives. A common goal of the people I meet is to be able to get down on the floor and play with their children or their grandchildren; and of course, then be able to get up again. They want to be there for those same children and grandchildren—to know that they have a better chance of being around for them, watching them grow up and being with them during those wonderful times in their lives. They want to be free of embarrassment. Free of the fear of sitting on a chair and breaking it. Free to ride in an airplane and not have to use a seat belt extender. They also want to be free to walk down the aisle of an airplane, knowing that the people already sitting aren't praying that you won't sit down beside them.

Nobody chooses to live a life like that. Every morbidly obese person I have ever met has struggled with dieting just as much as I did. We have reached the point of desperation. There was a study done in the '70s by Dr. George Blackburn, who is an internationally recognized expert on obesity and clinical nutrition. He's currently at the Beth Israel Deaconess Hospital in Boston; and he's also at Harvard. In the '70s, Dr. Blackburn was interested in studying nutrition and the subject of starvation. Dr. Blackburn needed subjects to study in this field and placed a newspaper ad asking for people willing to starve. He was amazed that so many people volunteered; and even more amazed that many of the volunteers were overweight or obese. He starved the volunteers, but fed them just enough protein to maintain their muscle mass. The volunteers lost weight; yet when the experiments were over, the volunteers begged to continue with the program. They were willing to do anything, including starving, to lose weight.

Wright

Goodness. Could you tell our readers how illnesses are affected by weight loss?

Thompson

The most dramatic reversal of health problems is with Type II Diabetes. Eighty-two percent of those having weight loss surgery are cured of their diabetes soon after their surgery, according to research reported by Dr. Phil Schauer in the *Annals of Surgery*. Seventy percent of those with high blood pressure are able to stop taking medication.

Wright

You're kidding.

Thompson

No. Eighty percent of patients will develop normal cholesterol levels within two to three months following surgery. And there is significant improvement, if not cures, of asthma, sleep apnea, acid reflux, and stress incontinence. There is also significant improvement with arthritis and back pain because you're putting less weight and stress on your joints. It's a life saving operation.

Wright

I was fascinated by the circumstances leading to your decision to lose weight, especially the questions your nutritional physician asked you. Could you share that story with our readers?

Thompson

I had discussed my weight problems with my family physician several times, and he had reached his point of frustration with not being able to help me through dieting. So, he referred me to a nutritional physician who, after a brief exam, asked me a question that no one had ever asked me before. He asked me how much weight I wanted to lose. I thought that was a curious question. Don't we all approach dieting with the thought that "today, I'm going to go on a diet and will continue successfully on that diet until I lose all of my excess weight?" It is our expectation that we can then go off the diet and be slim and happy. He explained to me that losing weight did not work that way. He explained the following statistics to me. He said that if I dieted and were successful, the most I could expect to lose would be 5 percent of my weight. At 264 pounds, that would mean the best I could do through dieting alone was to lose 13 pounds. I wasn't happy with that prospect.

He then said there was another option. That option involved dieting, exercise, and taking a diet drug. Again, if I were successful, the most I could expect to lose was 10 percent of my weight. That was even worse because it involved exercise. With a herniated disc, I always associated exercise with pain. A 10 percent weight loss was only 26 pounds. I would still weigh 238 pounds. He did say there was a third option. He explained to me that if I hoped to be of normal weight, since I was morbidly obese, that my only chance was to have weight loss surgery. With that surgery I could lose 50 to 80 percent of my excess weight. I'd been fighting against statistics all my life with dieting. He also explained that the surgery was endorsed by the National Institutes of Health that set guidelines on who is eligible to have the surgery and who is not. Being morbidly obese, I qualified. Even though, I was shocked that despite all my struggles I had failed so miserably in controlling my weight, I was still intrigued by the idea and success of the surgery. It was not something that I rushed into, but I studied it and I gave it very serious consideration before I made my decision.

Wright

You know, to actually choose surgery for weight loss is certainly a major decision. What were some of the fears you were dealing with in order to make an informed decision?

Thompson

My first fear was not surviving the surgery. Any surgery is a risk, and the risk with that particular surgery is one death in 200 surgeries. Considering the generally poor health of those having the surgery, this number is surprisingly low. I also feared what my life would be like after the surgery. Eating is a central part of our existence. We celebrate by eating. Holidays involve eating. There are business lunches and parties. We eat when we're happy, and we eat when we're sad. Our ethnic cultures and our nationalities are identified by our food. I feared giving all of that up. I feared that I would never be able to eat normally again. But I was willing to give up eating "normally" to obtain a normal weight and a normal life. And as it turns out, I now eat like a normal-weighted person. I have control over what I eat. And I actually enjoy eating more now than ever because I control my eating. Food no longer controls me.

Wright

You've stated that you've been overweight for 20 years. During that time, you had tried many diets. The results of your diets seemed to always be the same. Initially you lost weight, but each time you regained the weight plus additional pounds. How do you account for all of those additional pounds?

Thompson

There are many biological reasons for obesity. Researchers, the National Institutes of Health, and the World Health Organization agree with those biological reasons. In fact, the World Health Organization has listed obesity as a disease since 1979. The insurance industry and the U.S. food industry do not agree. They approach obesity as a matter of personal responsibility. But researchers are convinced that our weight is controlled by a system of hormones, proteins, neurotransmitters, and genes that work together to tell the body how to store fat. And once weight is gained, it is the body's natural inclination to hold onto that weight. When you diet, the body resists starvation and weight loss as a means of preserving the species.

Those of us who are morbidly obese have that biological system which resists weight loss even more. If we were in hunter-gatherer days, we'd be at an advantage. We would be the ones to survive, while the thin members of the species died off. But living in the 21st century with fast food, computers, and automobiles, has put us at such a disadvantage that our health suffers. It's not a matter of simply eating less and exercising more, it's a disease. Telling me to lose weight was like telling someone with asthma to just breathe better. Genetics play a very significant role in obesity. You'll often see an obese parent who has obese children or all of the adult sisters in a family will be obese. That's very common. They share the same genetic tendencies toward obesity.

But let me tell you about my daughter. My daughter is 17-years-old. I was very blessed to be able to adopt her when she was 8-days-old. I have been the role model for my daughter. I have taught her about nutrition and set the example for her on how to eat, yet my daughter is very thin. She did not inherit my genes. I could make my daughter's favorite food, put it in front of her, and she would eat and stop. I would ask her if she was all right or if she didn't like the food;

and she would look at me with a puzzled look on her face and tell me that she was "full." And I would look back at her equally puzzled and wonder what "full" was because "full" was not something that I experienced. I was always hungry.

Wright

Now that your weight is under control and outwardly you are a new and thinner person, do people treat you differently than before?

Thompson

Yes, they do. That's partly because of how people approach those who are obese, as well as how I feel about myself. There's no doubt that I feel better about myself. I'm more outgoing, more confident, and I like myself better. When we like ourselves better, we are naturally more attractive to others. It's also human nature to avoid people who are failures. We all want to be associated with people who are successful. We all have failures in our lives. Some of us have failures with a job, some have marriages that could be better, or we might have a troubled child. All of these failures can be kept personal and private. But when we fail with our weight, that failure is there for everyone to see. It is there for everyone to judge us on. That's a crushing blow to the heavy person's self esteem.

Wright

For our readers who are considering weight loss surgery, as well as those obese people who are concerned about their weight, what advice could you share that might make their decision better and more informed?

Thompson

If you're overweight and don't qualify for the surgery, then diet, exercise, and medication are the options, bearing in mind that your object is to lose only ten percent of your weight. When you reach that goal, stop dieting and stabilize your weight. If you have additional weight to lose, work on maintaining that weight loss for a number of months; and then, begin again on another ten percent. The tabloid diets that claim you'll lose 15 pounds in 15 minutes are the worst avenue to take. They will only worsen your weight problem. Also, understanding how your body resists losing weight can help you through those discouraging plateaus. If you're to the point of morbid obesity, your only chance of being of normal weight is weight loss surgery. But even the surgery is not a guarantee. During the first year, you're in weight loss heaven as the pounds melt off. When your appetite returns, it becomes more difficult and you have to exercise control. But you have the tool of having a very small stomach to help you. So whereas before it was impossible, now it's manageable.

Wright

Before we finish this interview, do you have any thoughts that you would like to add, to share with our readers?

Thompson

It is important that society starts to recognize that obesity is a disease that is very common in adults and is becoming more prevalent in our children. This generation of parents will be the first to experience their children dying before them because of the health problems associated with childhood obesity. When obesity is recognized as the disease it is, the social stigma will lessen and more research and treatment options will become available. Since 1985, the number of morbidly obese Americans has increased from one in 200 to one in 50. We need to work proactively to reverse this trend. We'll not be a healthy society until this problem is faced as the disease it is.

Wright

Today, we've been talking to Barbara Thompson. Barbara, it's been such a pleasure. I really appreciate you spending this much time with us in this interview; and I can't tell you how much I've learned. So, thank you so much for being with us on *Conversations on Health and Wellness*.

Thompson

Thank you very much, David, it was my pleasure.

About The Author

Barbara Thompson is a consultant, speaker and author in the field of obesity and weight loss surgery. Her book, *Weight Loss Surgery, Finding the Thin Person Hiding Inside You,* is termed the "unofficial bible among bypass patients" by the *Philadelphia Inquirer.* Barbara dieted her way to morbid obesity and facing disability she underwent gastric bypass surgery in 2000. Now at normal weight, Barbara has maintained a 125 weight loss since her surgery. She understands life from both ends of the scale and is sought after as a speaker nationally on obesity, bariatrics and weight loss surgery.

Barbara Thompson

WLS Center, Inc.

488 Diablo Drive

Pittsburgh, Pennsylvania 15241

Phone: 877-440-1518

Email: Barbara@wlscenter.com

www.wlscenter.com

Chapter 5

RICHARD TYLER

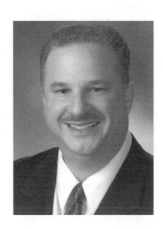

THE INTERVIEW

David E. Wright (Wright)

Today we're talking to Richard Tyler. Richard is the CEO of Richard Tyler International, Inc., an organization named one of the top fifty training and consulting firms in the world. Mr. Tyler's success in sales, leadership, management, quality improvement, and customer service, and his reputation for powerful educational methods and motivational techniques have made him one of the most sought after consultants, lecturers, and teachers. Mr. Tyler shares his philosophies with millions of individuals each year through keynote speaking, syndicated writing, radio, television, seminars, books and tapes. Mr. Tyler's book, *Smart Business Strategies: The Guide to Small Business Marketing Excellence,* is being hailed as one of the best books ever written for small business marketing. His philosophies have been featured in *Entrepreneur Magazine* as well as in hundreds of articles and interviews. Mr. Tyler is the founder of The Leadership for Tomorrow, an organization dedicated to educating young adults to the importance of self-esteem, goal setting, and lifelong success. He also serves as a board member to such community organizations as Be An Angel, a non-profit organization helping multiple handicapped and profoundly deaf children to have a better life. Richard Tyler, welcome to *Conversations On Health And Wellness*!

Richard Tyler (Tyler)

Thank you, David. I am absolutely delighted to be here.

Wright

What have your years of experience as the CEO of a successful international management, training and consulting firm taught you about wellness?

Tyler

This business has taught me so many different things for sure. But interestingly, I learned some of the most valuable lessons about wellness when I was a young man involved in competitive activities. I was fortunate to have achieved success in high school mainly due to intensive physical training, but after high school, the competition kept improving. My physical strength alone wasn't enough. I very quickly learned that I had to do more. I started focusing my attention, most of my attention, on mental wellness as well as having physical wellness. So getting prepared mentally for each contest actually became more important than the physical preparation. But it was the powerful combination that allowed me to achieve my goals. One key and critical thing in preparing mentally is that I found out that your mind doesn't care whether you're going to be a success or failure. It will do whatever it is that you program it to do, whatever you condition it to do. Therefore creating a wellness program for your mind is critical in achieving success, and it's critical in keeping your body and mind healthy.

Wright

How has that lesson helped you in your professional career?

Tyler

The focus on health and wellness as a state of attitude is really central to all of the training programs that we offer at Richard Tyler International, Inc. We teach a concept called the *Tyler Learning Six*, which serves as a framework for focusing students on the mental conditioning necessary to achieve success. The effective application of this framework will not occur without the appropriate mental wellness.

Wright

Why do you believe mental wellness is so important to achieving success?

Tyler

Because I believe that all aspects of wellness—spiritual, emotional, physical, and mental—are connected. In other words, there is a universal synergy between them. When any one of those is disconnected, the individual loses effectiveness in the ability to meet his or her potential. I also believe that there are no shortcuts to lasting success. Success happens when there is a commitment to excellence, a commitment to continuous improvement, a distain for the status quo, and the resolve to never be satisfied. But you will never get a real commitment if you don't have the right mental state of being.

Wright

So how do you teach mental wellness?

Tyler

Well, again it starts with commitment. We ask our students to pledge their commitment to fully engage in our education programs. Once a part of any of our programs, the students are provided with a wide variety of practical techniques that must be understood and practiced to be effective. One aspect of our success philosophy is to introduce a new language. This new language really begins to re-shape how students speak and how they think. For example, we teach our students to recognize what I call "Power Positive"™ words, words like "breakthrough," "discovery," "innovation," and "new." We teach them to distinguish between fear words and excellence words. Fear words are words that create psychological fear within them or psychological fear with their customers, clients, spouse or children. Words like "contract" or "cheap" or "problem" have a negative impact on the listener and they should be replaced with excellence words like "agreement" or "value" or "opportunity" or "challenge." We teach our students to use "Anchors"™ and "Testers"™ and those are particular types of language that we use to identify methods in the communication process. We teach them to be careful of words we call "Qualifiers"™ or soft words like "try," "maybe" and "might." You know, I'll give you a quick example of this if I may, David.

Wright

Sure.

Tyler

Imagine if you and I were on a plane and we were flying across the country. I'm sure you've flown many times, haven't you?

Wright

Yes.

Tyler

So we're flying across the country and it was a terrible flight. It was turbulent and we were bouncing all over. It was so bad that the flight attendants were not able to even give us a soft drink or wait on us in any way. We're about a hundred miles out of where we're going to land, and the pilot comes on and says, "I want to thank you for flying Tyler Airlines today. We appreciate your business. We know you had a choice of carriers and we appreciate your coming onboard with us. We apologize for the fact that we weren't able to give you any in-flight service, but your safety and the safety of our flight attendants is our primary concern. Again, I want to thank you for flying Tyler Airlines and I just want to let you know I'm going to 'try' to land this plane safely."

Wright

Oh my!

Tyler

Well, you're laughing, right?

Wright

You had me until you said "try."

Tyler

I did. Now let's think about that for just a second, David, because that word "try" is used throughout our language. It permeates everything we do. Now this is just one example of a soft word or "Qualifier"™. But if I said that in that flying circumstance, what would you be thinking?

Wright

Oh my goodness!

Tyler

"You'd be thinking, "What do you mean *try* to land this plane safely, you had better land this plane safely." And you be thinking, "I'd better check out those crash instructions that I didn't pay any attention to when I first got on the plane." But let me tell you what really just happened. What happened is that "try" doesn't mean anything different than it always means except for in that moment, in that context, I put it in a life or death circumstance. So what happened was your subconscious mind, which knows what "try" means all the time, took it and when I said, "try to land this plane safely," it shoved what "try" really means forcefully right through into the conscious mind. It said, "Hey, wait a minute! This guy might not land this plane safely!" You see? So all of a sudden its real world, real impact was noticed by you. Well, it has the same impact on us psychologically at the subconscious level all the time, when we say, "Well, we'll try this new product or we'll try that new method or I'll try to do my best." What we've really programmed our mind to do mentally is accept failure. We said to ourselves, "Hey, if it doesn't work, it's okay because we're just giving it a try." Some people will say, "Well, you can't be positive on every single thing. You can't say I'm going to do this." No, you don't have to say you're going to do it.

Well, let's back up a second. You really do have to condition your mind to think it. Does that mean there's a chance for failure still? Absolutely. When you got on that plane, David, you knew that that plane could come down. You knew that there was a potential out there that it might crash, but you still got on and you didn't think about that because you thought about where you wanted to go. The desire to get where you wanted to go was more important than the initial fear or trepidation that you had of that remote possibility the plane would go down. Well, you have to do the same thing in conditioning your mind. You have to condition it the same way to believe that the likelihood of failure, that you can't resolve and learn from and move on from, is slim to none and you're going to make adjustments along the way. Because see, failure really only occurs when you stop making adjustments toward success. That's where real failure occurs. So, little words like "try," "might," "maybe" and "could" permeate our language. I hear so many people who wonder why they are not being more successful, and they say sentences like this: They say,

"Well, you know, I'm going to give it my best shot. I'm going to give it a try and if I work really hard, well maybe I might possibly be successful." You hear what I'm saying there, David?

Wright

Oh yeah.

Tyler

There's not any likelihood that this individual is going to be a success. They're going to have to stumble into success. Anytime you stumble into success, it doesn't sustain itself a long time. The process that we use in our training program gets people focused on their attitude as well as the message that they are sending. Ultimately, it works to improve a person's success personally and professionally. Of course, it also gives an organization a common language so that people are communicating more effectively with each other rather than having a hodgepodge system or methodology. I'm talking about all of the words that we give them, all of the language, all of the processes we put in place, not just the Qualifiers™ or soft words we were talking about with "try." That brings a team together and whether they're all under one roof, whether they're spread across the country, or whether they're stretched out across the world on several continents, they have a common language, a common methodology, and a common process. It reduces rework and creates success and confidence. Once this happens you significantly impacted a corporate culture, and corporate culture is the single biggest factor that drives success in any organization. When I say success, I'm talking about not just financial success, I'm talking about satisfaction from customers, which leads to financial success, and I'm talking about moral and ethical success as well. A corporate culture has to be driven within moral and ethical boundaries and that's critical in mental health and wellness.

Wright

Without using the word, the two worst fear words as you've just used, I was listening when you said the word "problem" as being a fear word. We had a fellow come into our company a few months ago and change our language. You know when someone was asking us to do things we'd say, "No problem." He kept saying never use that again. Always say things like, "I will be more than pleased to do that for you. I will be happy to do it for you," those kind of words.

Tyler

Well, absolutely. What he was doing was conditioning you with a positive response.

Wright

Right.

Tyler

And although "no problem" may not in itself cause failure, it's not usually a single thing, David, that creates an environment of failure or lack of strength in mental health and wellness, it is the collection of all the little things that add up.

Wright

Right.

Tyler

When you think of a person that has a heart attack because their arteries are closed, it's not a single piece of plaque attaching itself to the artery that causes the heart attack. It's the one piece on top of the one on top of the one on top of the one, until the artery is finally closed, then the person has a heart attack.

Wright

So if you teach this methodology in mental wellness, how well received is the prospect of a corporate culture change?

Tyler

In most organizations it's exceedingly well received. We call that portion of the program Neuro-Success Conditioning™, in other words, the conditioning of our minds towards success. Remember we offer comprehensive education programs in sales, management, leadership, customer service, quality improvement, and each of those wraps around a Neuro-Success Conditioning™ component. That's part of our corporate culture and it is exceeding well received in the organizations that want to create and sustain success. You know, it's an interesting thing that you bring that up, David, because sometimes what happens is that the leaders of the company may know something needs to take place. But they don't think that their people are going to want to buy into that corporate change. "So they think, gee, do we really want to go in this direction?"

One of our clients recently was in a circumstance such as this and they asked us to assist the management in their organization to create a corporate culture change, but they were really hesitant that they were going to get buy in from their folks. They thought that their people were just not going to be excited about the prospects of education and development and improvement of their own minds and their own attitudes, their own beliefs and philosophies, enhancing those types of things. So I said, "You've got a national sales meeting coming up, why don't you let me do a Keynote speech before we introduce the education programs. Let me speak to the group and tell them what the program's all about and lets talk to them about success. We'll talk to them about mindset. We'll talk to them about the types of things that create wellness in the mind and in the body and in a business because they all have to be connected in one way, shape, or form. So they agreed to that. I spoke to two different groups. Two groups that they were absolutely certain were going to be hesitant. Hesitation is a natural thing when you're walking into an uncertain area. As a matter of fact, it is instinctive for us.

Wright

Right.

Tyler

It's part of our survival instinct. We have to sit back and say, "Oh, is this the right way to go?" If we hadn't done that, if our ancestors hadn't done that, you and I wouldn't be around having this conversation today. But hesitation that causes no action to take place is not good. So we have to learn to control and direct those instincts. Well, I have to tell you that when I finished each talk, only forty-five minutes to each one of the groups, the results were amazing. These groups that management thought were going to be negative and not excited about a corporate culture change towards education, cost improvement, and improvement of the mind, responded by giving me a standing ovation. In each session there were well over a hundred people from that particular division of the company. Their enthusiasm has continued to grow along with more business and more success stories. Individuals from this company who have gone through our on-going program ended up talking about life changing experiences for them as it relates to how they became more successful in sales and more successful in leadership by learning how to control their attitude and their mind. Now of course we're teaching them sales techniques and management techniques as well.

Wright

You teach an Immersion™ Program that I understand is quite intense. Can you tell us about that?

Tyler

We have several different types of Immersion™ Programs, and yes, they are all intense. By the nature of the name 'Immersion'™, it does exactly that. It immerses the student in the learning process. I have found that people can learn primarily two different ways. I am speaking primarily about an education program. They learn by spaced interval repetition, which is a small amount of information. Then you go away for a while and you get to work with it a little bit and then you come back, and so forth, learning a little more each time. Now there's always some loss of information in that process. With the spaced interval repetition, the part that is the biggest challenge is that you never get the whole picture until you're all the way at the end. So you can't always implement the philosophies, strategies and techniques because you may not have all you need to know for quite some time. So I decided that I wanted to <u>ramp</u> success up with individuals and corporations faster. So I pioneered the development of Immersion™ Programs in sales, management, leadership, executive strategies, and so forth. They are very intense, very powerful, very results oriented programs.

Let me give you an example. Our Sales Immersion™ Program is one in that series and it's seven days long. Each day can easily be twelve to fifteen hours. The program's designed for those who are ready to commit to achieving excellence in their personal and professional lives. It's not for the weak of heart. The program teaches basic principles as well as fundamental success techniques. But you have to want to be there. You have to want to be committed. We conduct these in remote conference center locations where there are no distractions. There is no leaving the campus. It's not a party environment. It's an intense learning environment and when people leave at the end of that week, or if it's our management program it's a fourteen day program, they have a practical set of skills and attitudes and beliefs that they can put into play right away. Now those skills will still need to be built upon and honed and refined and nurtured and cared for in their use so that they become habits, but at the same time they've got a full fledged set of skills that they can walk away with and put to use immediately. Whether it be in leading people, whether it be in managing people, whether it be in sales, we take practical experiences and we plug them into the class where people can be successful in areas they are currently working on.

We also have many other components in an Immersion™ Programs. We have creativity involved. You know, David, one of the things I found in the last number of years is creativity is gone in many places. Individuals have lost their ability to creatively think or they believe they don't have the ability to creatively think. To rekindle this ability we put them into environments where they have to creatively think to be successful. Something else about our Immersion™ Program that is unlike every other training and education program that's out there for corporations or for individuals is attendance does not give you a graduation certificate. In other words, when you attend, you're tested throughout. You're tested in written form. You're tested in presentation skills; everything that we're teaching gets tested orally and in writing and presentation form. There's team situations that there are group grades on. There are situational role-plays that involve group grading as well.

So there are many, many, many aspects and levels that are taught and in order to pass, a student must have a 90% grade point average. Some folks would say to me, "Well, 90%, that's very difficult, isn't it?" Of course it is, however we're there along the way to coach them and give them whatever assistance they need to help them to get that 90% grade point average, David, keep in mind we're talking about a commitment to excellence, not a commitment to good and not a commitment to average. You cannot be ultimately successful, and I'm not talking just financial success, I'm talking personal success, personal health, personal mind well being and business success. That can't happen without dedication and drive. By the nature of the word "commitment" as I define it, it is no matter how difficult, no matter how stressful, no matter how uncomfortable, you're going to go through the actions. So, sure a 90% grade point average is difficult. Virtually all the students end up passing even though many of them think they are not going to pass. They reach within themselves and they achieve things that they didn't think that they could achieve. By achieving those things that they didn't think they could achieve, what do you think happens to their self-esteem?

Wright

It has to sky rocket.

Tyler

Of course. I have learned that nobody, *nobody*, ever performs above their personal level of self-esteem for very long. So raising your self-esteem is critical to improvement and success.

Wright

Right.

Tyler

The greater a person's self esteem is the more they are going to achieve and the stronger their mental state of mind.

Wright

Is there a mental conditioning aspect to this Immersion™ strategy?

Tyler

Oh, absolutely. I mean make no mistake that there's a great deal of material to cover in a short period of time, but more importantly, students are learning a mental conditioning regiment that becomes a necessary component of their success. I often remind people that achieving success requires a mental determination to do whatever it takes within moral and ethical boundaries—and that's very important to get the desired outcome. The indoctrination of success principles often requires a student to do some rewiring. That doesn't happen automatically. It takes some conditioning. We push the students hard, but the results are tremendous, and when people come out of the program, they say it is one the most exciting, most invigorating experiences they've had in their life. The short and long term results people achieve verify that.

Wright

What do you find to be the biggest impediment to staying mentally healthy?

Tyler

One of the most powerful forces of nature, the status quo. You know, given the choice, most people take the easier way. It's hard to make changes. It's easy to leave things the way they are. There are plenty of programs out that that will convince people that they can have unlimited success with little or no effort. We make it clear that we don't offer any shortcuts to success. We just don't believe they exist and we don't waste time, anyone's time, pretending to offer one. Our students learn very quickly that excellence requires commitment, that mental determination to accept only excellence no matter how difficult, not matter how uncomfortable, no matter how stressful. We give students the tools they need to succeed, but learning to use them requires hard work. And the education and hard work must be continuous. When students understand this and they want to engage in the learning process, excellence is the result.

Wright

In addition to the training programs you described, what other resources do you provide your customers to strengthen their mental wellness?

Tyler

Our customers learn the value of on-going refresher training and they believe in our philosophy of continuous development. That keeps our connection with our customers very strong. We also keep connected through our various book series, our audio programs, our *Excellence Edge Newsletter*™ and my TylerTips™ online newsletter. The TylerTips™ newsletter provides subscribers with no-nonsense, hard hitting, immediate actionable tips and techniques for staying sharp in achieving excellence in their business. Our connection in the various different ways with clients allows us to keep their mental attitude strong. Also a unique service that we offer is that anyone who attends one of our programs knows that for the rest of their lives, as long as we exist, they can pick up a telephone, they can send us an e-mail, tell us a challenge that they are having, and we get back to them. Inevitably, we get back to them in forty-eight hours. So many of our clients use us constantly to bounce off challenges that they may be having career wise, challenges they may be even having at home.

As a matter of fact, we just handled a career situation yesterday with a gentleman who called me up and said, "Hey, here's what's happening in my career. Here's some choices I'm thinking of making and I want to make sure that I've gone through the whole regimen in my head of what I should do and how I should do it. I was wondering if you could take a few minutes to go over it with me." We have clients that go back fifteen years who numerous times a year will contact us with various different situations. And David, once a student enrolls in one of our Immersion™ Programs, for the rest of their life, they can come back to a refresher and the investment is only 15% of the current tuition.

So year in and year out, we have people who come back. I can think of one VP of Sales of a company who comes twice a year. He uses Immersion™ as his mental conditioning and toughness regiment, to get the garbage out, get back into it to refocus. Two times a year he comes back and goes through the same program because he says it's the best investment he's ever made in his life. I should mention that although he is attending the same program, he learns new information at each. This is for two primary reasons. One is that every program has the personality of the students. So new input and challenges exist with each class. Second, we are constantly evaluating, adding and enhancing each program.

Wright

Is there a particular product or service that differentiates your business?

Tyler

What differentiates our business is our philosophy of the commitment to excellence. It's integrated into every single thing that we do. Our focus is on helping our customers understand how important mental wellness is to total health and total wellness, and of course, where personal responsibility fits into that. The techniques and skills that are necessary to achieve success require a commitment to lifelong learning and continuous improvement. I've seen it over and over. Commitment to excellence in your life, relationships, business, they'll all improve if you just make that commitment. The stronger the commitment, the bigger the improvement.

Wright

I think one of the problems that I have in all of the books on excellence is that excellence is really not defined as excellence. It sounds to me that you are closer to it and, you probably have nailed it. I like the idea of...I mean I would hate to go to a fourteen or fifteen day training course that was entitled "Whatever Excellence," and pass it with an eighty-five. You know what I mean?

73

Tyler

It doesn't make much sense, does it?

Wright

I mean, that's really not excellence.

Tyler

No, it really isn't and you have to remember there are a lot of people who look to fool people into believing that they can achieve great results with little effort.

Now that we've talked about excellence I'm going to throw a monkey wrench in the works. We have commitment to excellence on our programs and everything that we do, but David, I don't even believe excellence is achievable. So somebody's going to say to me, "Well, wait a minute. How can you say all these things about excellence and you don't think it's achievable?" I say, "I don't think it's achievable because we live in a world that changes." If the mark stood still, if the target stayed in one place, then we'd be able to get to excellence all the time and stay there. But the fact is that business changes, relationships change, life changes, global conditions change. There's something always going on so the target is constantly moving.

So when I say commitment to excellence, I'm talking about a commitment to the pursuit of constant improvement and development, and to head in a direction of abundance that your creator wanted you to have. The ability to get out from within you what you are capable of. That's what mental well-being is all about. Mental well-being is the ability to know that you can achieve great things and then to set a course of action to achieve them. No one was destined to *not* achieve greatness. We're *all* destined to achieve great things. We're all destined to head on the road towards excellence, but the fact of the matter is that most people won't put together a system or a process or condition themselves to do it. Well, our goal is to help them to condition themselves to do it. We're very proud of that calling.

Wright

Well, what an interesting conversation. I'm going to have to go back and think a lot about what you've been talking about. I never...this is a unique chapter in a health and wellness book.

Tyler

Thank you, David. May I assume you enjoyed our conversation?

Wright

Absolutely, I never considered there would be no way that you could be healthy or well and not be mentally strong.

Tyler

When you think about it, how long can you maintain physical fitness without a strong mind?

Wright

Right.

Tyler

It just can't happen for very long. The mind is the most powerful tool that we have, and it determines physical well-being. It determines what we are able to do. Science has learned through studies over the last few years that when it comes to healing the body from sickness and disease, an individual's ability to believe they are going to get well plays as significant a part as any doctor treatment that they are taking. So physicians need to be able to assist their patients in mental toughness and putting up with the challenges that are going to be there. Letting patients know they can resolve these challenges is even more important for doctors today than it ever was. With the revelations that we've found in science that the mind can help the body in getting well having a well conditioned mind is critical.

Wright

I have seen that first hand. I am married to a cancer survivor.

Tyler

It is fantastic that your wife is a survivor. For that to happen, somewhere she made a determination she was going to get well.

Wright

Well, everybody that I know, including myself, thought she was going to die except her. She was the only one that didn't think that.

Tyler

Well, God bless her for having the faith and having the mental fortitude and toughness to do it.

Wright

Well, she taught me a lot of faith too.

Tyler

Isn't that great?

Wright

Today we have been talking to Richard Tyler who is the CEO of Richard Tyler International, Inc., an organization named one of the top training and consulting firms in the world. As we have found out today, there are probably a lot of reasons that's true, and one of those reasons, I think, is Richard Tyler. Thank you so much, Richard, for being with us today on *Conversations On Health And Wellness*.

Tyler

Thank you, David, and God bless you.

About The Author

Richard Tyler is the CEO of **Richard Tyler International, Inc.™** an organization named one of the top training and consulting firms in the world. Mr. Tyler's success in sales, quality improvement, management and customer service and his reputation for powerful educational methods and motivational techniques, has made him one of the most sought after consultants, lecturers and teachers. Mr. Tyler shares his philosophies with millions of individuals each year through keynote speaking, syndicated writing, radio, television, seminars, books and tapes.

Mr. Tyler's book "*SMART BUSINESS STRATEGIES*™, *The* **Guide to Small Business Marketing** *EXCELLENCE*" has been hailed as one of the best books ever written for small-business marketing. His philosophies have been featured in *Entrepreneur Magazine®* as well as in hundreds of articles and interviews. Mr. Tyler's successful books include: *Conversations on Success, Conversations on Faith, Conversations on Customer Service and Sales, Leadership Defined, Marketing Magic, Real World Customer Service Strategies That Work, Real World Team Building Strategies That Work, Real World Human Resource Strategies That Work.*

Mr. Tyler is the founder of the **LEADERSHIP FOR TOMORROW**™ an organization dedicated to educating young adults in the importance of **self-esteem, goal setting** and **life-long success.** He also serves as a board advisor and is past Chairman to **Be an Angel Fund**, a non-profit organization helping multiple handicapped and profoundly deaf children to have a better life.

Richard Tyler
Richard Tyler International, Inc.™
P.O. BOX 630249
Houston, Texas 77263-0249
Phone: 713-974-7214
Email: RichardTyler@RichardTyler.com
www.RichardTyler.com
www.TylerTraining.com
www.ExcellenceEdge.com
www.DiscEducation.com

Chapter 6

DOROTHY CAMPBELL, M.ED.

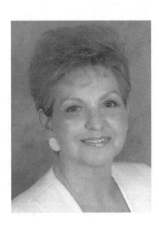

THE INTERVIEW

David E. Wright (Wright)

Today we are talking to Dorothy Campbell. Dorothy is the president of the Life Balancing Corporation and founder of the Life Cycle Institute and the Self Power Center where Body, Mind, and Spirit become ONE, a safe place for personal development and the discovery of self. She's the creator and presenter of Self-Power and Life Balancing classes, seminars, workshops, and keynote speeches. Her presentations guide individuals to take control of their body, mind and spirit, integrating these three aspects into one calm, healthy, happy being. Her teachings guide individuals on a journey of self discovery to bring balance, harmony & peace into their lives. Dorothy's enthusiasm and commitment motivate participants to put into practice the practical, easy to learn techniques and tools she shares in her presentations. She has more than thirty years of business experience, a Master's degree in Education, and is a National Guild of Hypnotists Certified Hypnosis Instructor. She is certified in Advanced Hypnotherapy, Neuro-Linguistic Programming (NLP), and Mind Body Therapy. She is a Usui and Karuna Reiki Master Teacher, a Life Balancing Therapy Master Teacher, Intuitive Dowser, a graduate of the Silva Method and the Open Doors School of Energy Healing, and a Personal Holistic Coach. Ms. Campbell is a

Personal Holistic Coach. Ms. Campbell is a speaker on the national level, is the author of *The Self-Power Newsletter*, and has written articles for several magazines. She has taught in the private sector and at numerous colleges. She's a member of the National Guild of Hypnotists, the American Association of Dowsers, and a charter member of the National Registry of Holistic Practitioners. Dorothy Campbell, welcome to *Conversations on Health and Wellness.*

Dorothy Campbell (Campbell)

Thank you, David. It's a pleasure to be speaking with you today.

Wright

How would you describe the work that you do now, and what is the purpose behind it?

Campbell

Well, David, I guess the answer to that question has many facets to it. My basic purpose is to guide individuals on their journey of self-discovery so that they can bring balance, harmony, and peace into their lives. Which, of course, we all strive for, but sometimes getting there takes some guidance, and that's where my work begins. I believe that the body, mind and spirit of a person must be looked at for their lives to really become in true balance. People come to me for assistance with challenges they are facing at the present time in their lives, whether it is physical, emotional, or spiritual. My work begins, David, with a discussion and a counseling session. We talk about what their challenges are at this point in their life, and then I explain each of the tools and techniques that I have to offer them. Together, we look at the physical, emotional, mental, and spiritual aspect and we decide on the appropriate modalities that will provide the most comfortable and effective solution. Since I offer so many resources that appeal to both the logical and ethereal minded individual, everyone can find a comfortable starting point from Self-Power training to Hypnosis, Holistic Coaching and then on to the healing modalities of Reiki, Life Balancing Therapy, and Dowsing. The clients that begin with the most logical teachings eventually become intrigued with the healing modalities and the possibility of being capable of doing self-healing.

Wright

Is what you do considered medical treatment? Does it replace conventional medical treatment or is it a complement to medical treatment procedures?

Campbell

That's a great question David. Nothing that I do is considered a medical treatment. I don't diagnose, nor do I prescribe. Everything that I do is a complement to medical treatments and procedures. The processes that I use address mainly the side effects of medication. I offer pain control, stress release, and calming effects while they are going through the necessary medical procedures. For example, I do sessions with and have a series of tapes for chemotherapy patients, cardiac recovery patients, child birth, and pre-operative and post-operative patients.

Wright

What does the medical profession think about this type of healing? Do you work with any medical professionals?

Campbell

The medical profession is becoming more receptive to the healing modalities that I offer. For some time now, they have accepted the body-mind connection. Now we just have to get them in sync with accepting the aspect of the spirit in healing a person. If someone's belief system (their spirit) is not part of the process, there is a possibility that healing may not take place, even though everything medically has been done properly. There are even some hospitals in my area where my pre-operative clients can take the list of positive affirmations, I created for them, into the operating room. The anesthesiologist will repeat those affirmations to the patient as they are going under anesthesia. The results are just astounding. They use less anesthetic, therefore, they awake sooner, are more alert, heal faster, and are much more comfortable through the entire process.

Wright

You have a diverse background, how did you get started in Health and Wellness areas?

Campbell

Well, it wasn't completely deliberate on my part, David. I've always followed my inner voice, my intuition, my higher self. I guess even as a child, I felt that part of my purpose was to help people in some way. Even in the corporate world I found my purpose being fulfilled. I found myself giving people the "Dot Campbell 101" speech on how they could achieve whatever they felt they wanted or needed by just concentrating on the positive sides of issues. Sounds simple enough, but not always easy to do. However, those that practiced what I gave them, actually accomplished what they had set out to do both physically and mentally. In fact, I used those people as research for my master's thesis on Motivation in the Business World. I honestly believe David, that we have available to us every answer we need in our entire life. We just have to stop and be quiet long enough to hear the answers. Our whole society is built on movement. If you're not moving, you're not productive. My belief system says that is not true. If you can slow down long enough to go inside and *just be*, the answers will come to you.

Wright

Tell me, what is Self-Power training? Why did you create it and then, of course, the Self Power Center?

Campbell

The Self-Power training came after I got my masters in education. I decided that I wanted to teach evening classes for women and created a four-week course. This first course was called *Today's Woman: Being the Best You Can Be*. During the classes, women would tell me that the men in their lives should hear my teachings. That's when I opened the course to everyone and the title changed to *Self-Power, when Body, Mind, and Spirit become ONE*. As we went through the four-week course, people were getting in touch with who they were and where they were headed, on many levels. When I made it co-ed, it was a wonderful experience for both the men and women in the classes because we began to understand how our subconscious mind influences communication between men and women. I've had great responses from gentlemen who have seen an amazing positive turn around in their lives and their relationships.

My Self-Power method is really built on the subconscious mind process. The whole process and theory of Self-Power is that you can't control other people. Sometimes you can't even control the situations that you get into. But what you can control are your responses and reactions to those people and situations. Self-Power training, teaches you the tools and techniques to understand where your perceptions are coming from and how you can take control of your responses and reactions. All of our perceptions are created in our subconscious mind from everything we've experienced and learned throughout our whole life because our subconscious mind never forgets anything. It's all filed away in our subconscious. Although sometimes we have difficulty finding some of the files. It will bring things forward when we least expect it without any explanation. The good news is it never forgets anything; the bad news is it never forgets anything. And part of its job is to protect us. Sometimes it gives us fears to keep us from doing something without giving the "why" of it. I teach people what that process is about and how to control their responses in a positive way so that they create positive results in their life. Once they understand the process, they make incredible positive changes. My book entitled, *A User's Manual for the Subconscious Mind* explains the process in very basic terms and offers easy-to-learn techniques to begin to use the subconscious mind as the incredible tool that it is. By using the information that I share in this book, it is possible to create the life that you truly want.

I established the Self-Power Center so there would be a safe place for people to come and explore their own development and find out who they are. It's a place where they can *just be*. Each student learns how to go within themselves and find out what's best for them. It has become an even more incredible place since we do our Reiki healing circles there periodically. So it is also an amazing healing environment for a lot of people.

Wright

What is a "Personal Holistic Coach" as compared to personal coaches, or life coaches that seem to be everywhere?

Campbell

I became a personal coach in the early '90s to assist my Self-Power students that still needed help. At the time, the word wasn't very prolific and everybody thought I was some kind of a sports coach. The more people I coached, the more I realized that I was dealing with many different aspects of their lives, even into their spiritual belief system. That's when I added the word "holistic" to the coach title. My purpose is to assist the whole person, in all aspects of themselves and their lives. I believe that if you don't address all of the aspects of a person's being, it's not complete. There's not balance there.

Wright

I noticed that you often refer to the subconscious mind in your writings. How does the subconscious mind fit into the work you do and how did you become interested in it?

Campbell

I have always been fascinated with the subconscious mind process. I guess I've studied it for most of my life. A lot of my Self-Power teachings are based on the process that the subconscious mind takes us through each time that we encounter a person or situation. That subconscious mind process is a big part of the healing work, David, because what you believe, you think, and what you think, you become. So, reprogramming the perceptions of the subconscious mind is a major part of all of my work. We all have a subconscious mind, we are born with it. It's there all the time and it's an amazing tool once you understand how to utilize it. And it doesn't cost anything. It's there for all of us to use without any charge and the positive results that you can produce with it are absolutely phenomenal. The hypnosis, the pain control, the stop smoking, and all of the aspects of hypnosis are based on the subconscious mind process. So much of what we think and do initiates in our subconscious mind. My belief that "we become what we think" is what led me to write my book on the subconscious mind's process.

Wright

What is hypnosis? I have been on cruise ships where people get up and cluck like chickens and it's hilarious. But what is it and how does it work?

Campbell

Hypnosis is actually focused attention. For example, have you ever been driving down a highway that you drive all the time to get home, and you miss your exit?

Wright

Oh yes, many times.

Campbell

Okay, that's called "road hypnosis." You are so focused on your thought process that you totally miss the exit. That's what hypnosis does. It distracts your conscious mind, that chattering mind that's constantly making judgment calls on you. It's the rational part of you. Your subconscious mind is where you can do some reprogramming, some re-perception so that you can get to where you want to go. Hypnosis puts you into a very relaxed state. Your body and conscious mind feel comfortable and calm, while your subconscious is still completely aware of what is transpiring. Your just letting go and drifting into a place of calm and peacefulness, yet you may be aware of sounds around you. Ever been at a boring concert or event and doze off and then you jump because you wake up?

Wright

Unfortunately, yes.

Campbell

You where drifting into alpha, completely relaxed, but still aware enough that an increase in the volume of the sounds around you brought you back to complete awareness. Hypnosis takes you to that wonderfully calm, relaxed alpha state. You're no longer as aware of the outside sounds around you. You're just listening to the sound of my voice. Let me dispel a couple of things that most first-time hypnosis clients ask about, "Am I going to do something silly." You won't do anything under hypnosis that you wouldn't normally do after a few drinks, it just kind of puts your inhibitions aside. If you always wanted to be an entertainer and I tell you to get up on the table and dance like Elvis, then you'll do it. If you truly have no desire to perform in front of an audience, then you won't do it. The other thing people are concerned about is that if something happens to me, are they going to be hypnotized for the rest of their life. If I stop talking for any length of time, you will either fall asleep and wake up normally or you will just come out of hypnosis. Hypnosis with a qualified, certified Hypnotist can assist you in accomplishing the goals that you truly want. It's one of the most amazing processes you can go through to create success in your life.

Wright

Tell me, what is Reiki and energy work?

Campbell

Reiki and energy work are wonderful healing modalities. Reiki and all energy work emanate from a higher source. We are all made of energy. Energy flows through us at all times. Energy workers train to connect to the higher energy source and direct it to an individual. Healing energy work has probably been in existence before man was capable of documenting it. The Bible speaks of healing with the "laying on of hands." Reiki is the name of one of the energy work systems. I believe that we all have the ability inside of ourselves to heal. Our bodies do not want to be sick, but we have lost the ability to help heal ourselves because we have this wonderful medical profession. We can just go to the doctor's office and get a pill. That was not done a long time ago. Our ancestors were more in tune with their bodies. They helped heal themselves with herbs, rest and prayer to return to well-being. Reiki to me is a very high form of prayer. Reiki is not a religion, even though it is spiritual by nature.

A basic translation of Reiki is, that it is life-giving energy from a higher source. Because this energy emanates from a higher source, it will go wherever it is needed to heal the client. My belief system is that due to the wisdom of its source, Reiki can do no wrong. Reiki is a non-intrusive technique that treats the whole person; body, mind and spirit.

During a Reiki session a client will experience feelings of relaxation, peace, security and well-being. They will feel surrounded by the loving, healing light of the Universe, as the energy flows through their entire being. It is truly difficult to put such an uplifting experience into words. However, once you have experienced the loving, healing, energy of Reiki, you will understand it more fully. Reiki can be a life-altering experience—but in the most positive, possible way.

As I already mentioned in our conversation David, I accepted early in my life that my purpose was to help others. Although I knew that my intuition, my spirit, was guiding me, I did not recognize until my introduction to Reiki, where my path was leading. Through Reiki, I have not only assisted others in improving the physical, emotional, mental and spiritual levels of their being, but have a greater understanding and acceptance of my purpose and the Universal Energy, God that placed me on this path.

That understanding of my purpose has allowed me to accept the guidance that was sent to me in creating my Life Balancing Therapy process. During a session, the client becomes totally calm as I talk them through a relaxation process. Then the healing Universal energy begins to flow through their body. Whatever their intention; to release unresolved issues, to gain insight and focus, or to just relax and be, this soothing, healing process manifests their intention into reality. Most clients, especially if it is their first time experience with Life Balancing, will comment on how "light" they feel, as though all the things that were weighing them down have been lifted. They leave feeling calm and very balanced.

Wright

What is dowsing and how does it fit into your work? Do you use it to locate water?

Campbell

Most people think of dowsing as finding water and there are a lot of great dowsers who are still called water wizards. Even today, some people make a good living dowsing for water. I use dowsing as an intuitive tool to teach people how to access their intuition using either a pendulum or dowsing rods. Because as human beings, we have to see something happening. They'll see the pendulum or the rods move and give them the answers that they need. Using dowsing tools that let them see that something is actually happening, allows them to begin to trust their intuition. I relate intuition to a muscle that is within our body, if you don't use it then it will become weak and of little use to you. But if you exercise that muscle on a regular basis, then it becomes stronger and will give you all the support that you require from it.

David, I believe that we are all born with intuition, a sixth sense. But few of us use this wonderful inherent gift to its full potential. This is due mostly to our deep involvement in the logical, material world and its influence on our daily lives that does not allow the time or encouragement to utilize this natural skill.

I believe that we each have access to all the answers that we require. We just need to get back in touch with that place that holds those answers for us. Dowsing is an ancient method of accessing the intuition to receive the answers and knowledge needed to fulfill a purpose.

I teach students how to locate, balance and expand the four basic energy fields around the body, and scan and energize the seven main chakra centers within the body to create a feeling of peace and well-being. David, allow me to explain. We have four basic energy fields outside of our bodies—physical, emotional, mental, and spiritual.

These energy fields need to be in specific order and approximately the same distance apart. When there is an imbalance in these fields our well-being is effected. The same holds true for the seven main chakras within the body. Chakra is the Sanskrit word for wheel. Chakras are "wheels" of rotating energy. The chakras guide the flow of energy through the physical body. The energy flow of a chakra can identify imbalance or stress. My students learn meditations and visualizations that assist in expanding and aligning both the four basic energy fields around the body and the seven main chakras within the body, to produce balance, harmony and peace within their entire being.

Wright

I understand that you built a labyrinth, a medicine wheel, and a meditation garden in your backyard.

Campbell

Yes, I have David. The labyrinth started out when I went to my first dowsing convention. I couldn't find the seminar that I wanted to go to, so I found the auditorium and sat down to review the list of upcoming seminars. I didn't realize until an instructor began to speak, that there was a seminar scheduled at that time in the auditorium. I didn't want to be a distraction, so I just sat there as the instructor began to explain labyrinths. Never having read much about labyrinths, I was totally fascinated with it. Each person was permitted to walk the labyrinth that was in the auditorium. The moment I got into the center of the labyrinth, I closed my eyes and I saw a labyrinth in my backyard. So I knew I had to build the labyrinth in my backyard. That was the message that I got. I had no idea why, David, I just knew that I needed to build that labyrinth.

That spring I built the labyrinth in my backyard. It is basically for my clients and my students. It is an amazing meditative path to walk. It is particularly helpful for those that find they have difficulty meditating due to conscious distractions. When you walk the labyrinth, your conscious mind is concentrating on walking and therefore doesn't bring as many other issues into your thought process. You are able to go within, meditate and receive the calm, peace or perhaps even answers to questions that you have. Unlike a maze, a labyrinth has only one path in and the same path out. There is only one way to walk a labyrinth and you can't get lost. Walking the labyrinth is sometimes called "Circling to the Center."

My labyrinth is a seven circuit labyrinth, a classic design which is the most widely found pattern. The seven circuits coordinate with the seven main chakras within the body. Each person's experience walking the labyrinth is unique, depending on their intent and where they are in their life at the time. Which also means that each time that you walk the labyrinth you may experience something different. A labyrinth walk may release unwanted feelings and issues or bring focus, clarity, peace, calm and contentment.

The labyrinth has many uses. Each individual creates their own intention for their walk. Many people use my labyrinth as a place to dump their problems at the end of the day. They stop by after work, go to the labyrinth and begin their walk. When they reach the center, they hold the intention to just leave all of their concerns there in the center of the labyrinth. They walk back to the entrance, go home a much calmer being and have a wonderful evening with their family.

Many of my students and clients were using the labyrinth on a regular basis and felt a loss when the heavy snows of New England made it impossible to walk the labyrinth. So I began to create finger labyrinths, small portable labyrinths that can fit easily in a purse or briefcase. I have one in a plastic case that the children seem to be drawn to. It seems like a game to them. But in truth, it is bringing them some balance and focus. As you walk a labyrinth and shift your direction, you also shift your awareness from right to left brain inducing receptive states of consciousness and focus. This process has been helpful with some ADD children for calm and focus.

Building the medicine wheel in my backyard came about in practically the same manner as the creation of the labyrinth. I was in Sedona, where I have had some amazing things happen to me. I went to a class and found that it had been cancelled. The facilitator asked if I would like to experience a walk on a medicine wheel instead. I accepted her offer. She took me to a medicine wheel that was built on one of the higher points in Sedona. Again, I had the same type of experience when I reached the center of the medicine wheel as I had at the center of the first labyrinth I walked. When I closed my eyes and asked for a message, the message I got was to build a medicine wheel in my backyard. When I came home that fall, there was a big pile of leaves in one spot in my backyard which I raked into the woods. About two days later, there was once again a pile of leaves on the exact same spot, which I again raked into the woods. The leaves just kept piling up in that same spot over and over again. So I took that as my sign, that's where the medicine wheel needed to be.

A wheel or circle has been a sacred symbol to many cultures over time. The importance is not the circle itself, but what it represents—change. The circle in the Medicine Wheel is used to represent the changing cycles. This could mean the seasons of life (birth, mid-age, old age)or the changes surrounding the development of projects. The word medicine does not refer simply to healing, but anything that promotes harmony with all creation is medicine. It is important to realize that the Medicine Wheel is about coming into harmony with the natural flow of life's changes, bringing balance to your entire being.

The Native North American medicine wheel uses 7 directions, the compass directions of north, south, east, west and also includes above, below and within. Each direction of the wheel has different qualities or aspects which are medicine for you when you walk the wheel. Each individual will be drawn to the direction that contains the medicine that they need for the day—energy for new projects and rebirth to the east—power and wisdom to the north—intuition and insight to the west—nurturing and peace the south. They allow their intuition to take them to what feels right for them.

The medicine wheel is walked a little differently than the labyrinth. Where the labyrinth has a specific path that you take walking to the middle and back, you enter the medicine wheel from the east direction, called the East Gate, where the sun rises. You begin walking the medicine wheel in a counter-clockwise direction three or more times to release all negativity. From this point on David, there are many methods to walking the medicine wheel. The most basic is to just allow your intuition to guide you on the path until you are drawn to stop. The direction of the compass where you stop on the medicine wheel will give you what you require for this particular walk. Before you leave the medicine wheel, always leaving through the East Gate where you entered, you should walk the wheel clockwise three or more times to reinforce the positive energy you have created while walking the medicine wheel.

The medicine wheel is also something that the children enjoy walking. They are so open and are guided easily by their intuition to walk the right direction and stop at the appropriate compass point for them. I created a tape to assist the adults in walking the medicine wheel, but the children don't seem to need any assistance, they just let their intuition lead them on their path.

David, the meditation garden was created between the labyrinth and the medicine wheel, so that people can sit down and meditate on whatever is processed in either one of these amazing walks. The meditation garden is another place where my students and clients visit on their own whenever they feel the need for a safe place to *just be.*

Wright

You spoke of great things that happened to you in Sedona. You take people on retreats to Sedona. How did you get that started? What do you do when you have them there?

Campbell

I started going to Sedona before I ever started any of this work. I have always felt so comfortable and at home there, that it became an annual trip for me. One year I took a friend with me and did a healing on her in the Boynton Canyon vortex. She had a rather large lump in her breast and was scheduled for a needle biopsy. She asked, "Can we get rid of it?" I said, "I sense that we can shrink it down so that it won't be so difficult for them to operate on." After I did the healing, I took a picture of where she had been lying down. When she went for the biopsy, they had to take her for a sonogram because they couldn't find the lump. When they found it, it was so small that instead of doing the needle biopsy, they just went in and took out the lump. The test results on the lump came back negative and she only had a couple of stitches from the procedure.

When we got the pictures developed, there was the most amazing picture of the energy coming down to where she had been laying. I got it enlarged and it has a place of honor in my sacred space, where I do all of my sessions. Well, David my students began noticing the picture and wanted to know the story behind it. When I explained to them what had happened, they decided that I needed to take them there. So the first trip started out as just taking a few students for a short visit. When we returned and they began telling everyone about the wonderful experiences that they had in Sedona and the vortex sites, I began getting calls asking when the next trip was scheduled.

Now I take groups there a couple times a year. While we're there, I take them to all the vortex sights. We do group meditations, individual meditations, and a lot of healing ceremonies. Every year I find something new that they can do. We have had Angel portraits and readings done, Indian fire ceremonies, drumming journeys, a flute concert in the middle of a red rock canyon. It seems David, every year something new is offered to me to pass on to the group that is traveling with me. Most important is that they receive many insights, clarity and the answers to their questions. Sedona is an amazing energy site where you can do a lot of clearing and releasing work and build up a reservoir of good positive energy to tap into after you arrive back home.

Wright

Many of our readers are going to be interested in health and wellness, and they are going to be prepared for some of the things that you've been talking about. They will be at different stages of belief levels in their lives. What do you say to those people that say some of these things that you've talked about in this interview have been out of their understanding. In other words, what do you say to those people who think that you are a couple of tacos short of the festival plate?

Campbell

That's nothing new or unusual. I've encountered that most of my life. I begin talking about their belief system and ask if they do believe in a higher power. I use the word "Universe" all the time, David, because I don't want to offend anyone's belief system, but to me the Universe is God. As long as they have a belief system in a higher power, I can begin to explain to them how all of the energy work actually processes. Prayer is part of energy work. With the energy work, you're connected in a different way to the actual prayer process. I may start out explaining logically. In fact, I think I mentioned to you that a lot of people start out very logically. They go through my Self-Power training and learn hypnosis, which for them is still a little bit on the logical side. Then all of a sudden, as we're talking about the subconscious mind, that process and their belief system, they begin to realize that they have believed these things all of their lives. It's just that they didn't want to talk about it. Now with me, it's okay to talk about it.

One of the great things about having the Center and another reason why I established it was to bring like-minded people together. I found after I took my first Reiki class, I had no one to talk to about what was transpiring in my spiritual life. As an officer in a financial corporation, discussing Reiki was not an acceptable topic of conversation. One of the purposes of the Center is to allow everyone that's working on these modalities to come in and talk about it so that they don't think they are out of the norm. We are becoming the norm. To heal yourself is normal. It's instinctive to want to make yourself better. Even as a child, if you bumped your knee, you grasp it with your hand. If you hurt yourself or you're crying, small children will come up and immediately want to put their hands on you and make you feel better. As human beings, it's normal from a very young age to give comfort this way and to try to heal people. We need to get back to that. We need to go back to those natural instincts that we have to offer nurturing and healing to ourselves and others.

If you look at the fact that we are spirits connected to a higher source, then there isn't anything that's outside of our condition. We have amazing abilities when we tap into our higher self, accept the possibilities and allow the process to happen. So, it's within your own belief system as to how or if you use all the inherent gifts you have been given to create a life of Harmony, Balance and Peace.

Wright

What an interesting conversation. I want to thank you, Dorothy, for being with us today and taking this much time to discuss what I consider to be a fascinating subject.

Campbell

Well thank you, David, for allowing me to share my insights about all the wonderful healing processes available to all of us and the amazing results that they offer.

Wright

Today we've been talking to Dorothy Campbell. She's president of the Life Balancing Corporation and founder of the Life Cycle Institute and the Self Power Center where Body, Mind, and Spirit become ONE, and as we have found today, knows what she's talking about and can help her clients. Thank you so much, Dorothy, for being with us today on *Conversations on Health and Wellness*!

Campbell

Thank you, David. It was my pleasure.

About The Author

Dorothy Campbell is a specialist in helping individuals take control of their body, mind and spirit to become ONE. She has a Masters Degree in Education and is currently completing her Doctorate in Metaphysics. She is a noted speaker, author, trainer, Holistic Practitioner and creator of numerous "one-ness" books and programs. Dorothy is President of the Life Balancing Corporation and founder of the Self Power Center. One of her numerous programs is to work with various medical professionals to facilitate a healing process that is both safe and comfortable for patients. Her mission is to light the path to attaining Balance, Harmony and Peace.

Dorothy Campbell, M.Ed.

Self Power Center

P.O. Box 516

Sharon, Massachusetts 02067

Phone: 781-784-7139

Phone: 877- 518-9464

Email: dorothyc@selfpower.net

www.selfpower.net

Chapter 7

JOANN MOTON

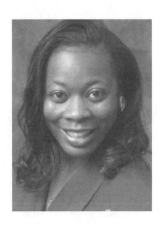

David E. Wright (Wright)

Today we're talking to Joann Moton. Joann is the Owner, and CEO of Confidence Unlimited, specializing in professional and personal development. The mission of her organization is to encourage, empower, and enable people to unleash their unlimited potential. Her presentations, services, and products are designed to promote holistic living. She presents information in a dynamic, unique, interactive, and entertaining manner to increase retention and usage. The slogan for her business and motto for her life is "Confidence unleashes the potential of unlimited power." Ms. Moton is a Certified Professional Trainer. Her services are designed to promote self-awareness and self-development. Joann Moton, welcome to *Conversations on Health and Wellness*!

Joann Moton (Moton)

It is a pleasure to talk to you today.

Wright

Joann, how would you define good health and wellness?

Moton

Wellness and good health mean taking proper care of your mind, body, spirit and soul. Let me explain what I mean when I use the terms mind, body, spirit, and soul. My definition and interpretation of these terms are based on the book, *Power of Purpose* by Clyde Odom.

"The body connects us to the physical world; it's our physical be-ing—the outer us. The soul comprises the intellect, the emotions, and the will of a person. It contains your personality, the part that makes you unique, makes you YOU—your past experiences, hurts, pains, joys." According to Drs'. Derek and Darlene Hopson, your soul also combines color, culture, history, and your essence. It contains expres-sion, resiliency, hopes, energy, conscience, dreams, and desires. The spirit is the part that communes with God. Our God consciousness.

The spirit communes with the spirit world, the spirit communes with our soul, our soul communes with our body. Good health and wellness mean doing things to prevent your body from illness and disease. This includes proper exercise and an active lifestyle. Taking in the right foods, nutrients and vitamins. Drinking plenty of water and getting the right amount of rest; treating your body right. Well-ness and good health also mean taking care of your spirit, mind, and soul. That is to say, growing spiritually—feeding your mind with positive thoughts, meditating, and nurturing your *self* are essential to good health and wellness. This includes working on your character flaws and working to develop strong positive personality traits. Your body is a temple. Put good things in it and good things will come out of it.

Wright

My temple has expanded through the years! What are your thoughts about dieting?

Moton

I don't like it very much. As a matter of fact, I don't like dieting at all. I actually consider it the big "D." When I hear the word "diet" it makes me think about foods that I cannot have, and they are usually the foods that I like most of all. I choose things I like, but just eat them in moderation. When I do overindulge I just turn up the big E, which is exercise.

Wright

Probably what you like in moderation is a lot better for you than some of the diet programs that I've been reading lately.

Moton

Yes, I do believe that eating foods in moderation is better than weight-loss diets. Many of the weight-loss diets and dietary products that are out these days have high contents of sodium, sugar or carbo-hydrates. So, when a great deal of these weight loss foods are eaten in excess they can be dangerous. Of course the key is checking with your doctor or health care provider before beginning any weight-loss pro-gram.

Wright

A lot of people now are talking about healthy lifestyle. What is your idea of a healthy lifestyle?

Moton

I think a healthy lifestyle is defined by the way that you live your life. It's not what you do occasionally, but what you do most of the time that counts. A healthy lifestyle means taking precautions to take care of your body, your mind, your spirit, and your soul; to take care of all parts of your life. Most people think of a healthy lifestyle only in terms of taking care of their body and they forget about the other components, which are our spirit, mind and soul. You cannot be healthy if you are always thinking negative thoughts or do not have any spiritual connection.

Wright

Down through the years I've probably lost about 1,000 pounds. Why doesn't dieting alone create long-term weight loss?

Moton

Dieting alone just doesn't work. You have all sorts of weight-loss diets; low-carbs, low-fat, low-cal, high-protein, etc. Usually, you follow these diets closely for a few weeks, a month, or until you lose the weight that you want to lose. But you're not going to stay on a diet for the rest of your life. Usually, when you stop dieting you start eating the same way you did before the diet; and then you gain all that weight back and then some. People think about reducing the intake of food, but they don't think about the other things that need to take place when you're trying to lose weight for the long-term. Exercise has to be built into that plan too. It goes back to actually changing your lifestyle and not just starving or depriving yourself of all the foods that you like. For me it's chocolate, I'm not giving it up!

Wright

I guess we all know that exercise has so many benefits. If we do know that, why don't more people do it?

Moton

Most people don't even like to hear the word exercise. When you think about exercise, it brings about unpleasant images. It seems too much like work. Just hearing the word makes you tired. If you think about it in this context, you will not want to do it. If you don't even like to hear the word exercise, you certainly will not want to do it. When you hear it, it makes you run the other way. So there needs to be a paradigm shift in the way we think about exercise. If you think about exercise as simply becoming more active by doing the things that you like to do such as: walking, biking, gardening and dancing, then you will enjoy it more. Yes, there is a need for some structured routine exercises too. Certain muscles need to be worked to develop and maintain tone, prevent osteoporosis, relieve arthritis and enhance the results you desire. Please don't fret, these too can be fun! Exercise with a partner. This helps you to be accountable and to encourage one another. Invest in some exercise tapes. You do have options. I power walk with weights, do some floor exercises, jump rope and hula-hoop daily. To me, these activities are fun. Have a variety of things you can do and move that body for a total of 30-45 minutes everyday. Don't just think of exercise as dragging yourself to the gym to sweat. You can have fun exercising.

Wright

I'd love to join you in that hula-hoop, but it's always down at my ankles. I can't ever seem to keep it going. I noticed, looking at your Confidence Unlimited client list, that some of your clients are churches. How can the church play a more active role in the health and wellness of its congregation?

Moton

Some of the churches are starting to minister to the whole person and not just the spirit. They are beginning to minister more to the mind, to the body, and the soul. Churches are starting to offer different resources and forums to the congregation in order to teach about health and wellness. Churches are now realizing that your soul and your spirit live inside a body and if the body isn't healthy you're not going to really feel like doing anything for the spirit. It's all connected. Churches are beginning to have health fairs and health forums, and are taking a more active role in making sure the congregation overall is healthy. I think that the church leadership, in promoting health and wellness to its congregation can take an even more active role. This can be done by leaders embracing a healthy lifestyle and speaking about the importance of taking care of the mind, body, spirit and soul. Teaching this principle based on scriptures would greatly help. Showing the congregation what the Bible states about taking care of the mind, body, spirit and soul would help as well. I believe this would make the congregation even more receptive to the resources and forums the churches are providing. Showing them scripturally how taking care of their mind, body, spirit and soul relates to worshiping God would help congregations take a more active role in holistic living; mind, body, spirit and soul.

Wright

I've noticed that people who have goals and a purpose in their life appear to be happier and healthier. Why do you think that is?

Moton

I believe that we all have to realize our purpose in order to be truly happy. I see many people that are surviving rather than living. They are struggling to get from one day to the next. They are just going through the motions with no true purpose. I believe that people who do not know their purpose are more depressed, have more illnesses, and encounter more unpleasant situations in their lives. These people feel no real excitement in their lives. However, when you do have a purpose, your life is full of excitement and focus. You have a sense of belonging; you live your life to the fullest, and you expect good things to happen to you. People with goals and purposes appear to have a more serene and comfortable life. This serenity is shared with others.

Wright

I talked today to a fellow named Dennis Brown, who lives in Texas and is a motivational speaker. His main drive is the difference between a good day and a bad day is your attitude. How much of a part does attitude play in health and wellness?

Moton

It's very, very important. I have heard that life is 10 percent of what happens to you and 90 percent of how you react to it. People with a positive approach to life live differently. I don't have a medical background and I am not a trained therapist, but I do observe a lot of people. I have also come in contact with many people in my business and have concluded that positive people appear to approach life in a more positive manner. They realize that life isn't always going to go the way they would like. They realize that you have to take the bitter with the sweet. In order to have lemonade you have to have the bitter lemons and the sweet sugar. In order to enjoy a rose you have to have the thorny thorns and the smooth petals. People with positive attitudes appear to take better care of themselves; mind, body, spirit and soul. In past years I have personally experienced the effects of a bad attitude. I felt bad, depressed—just down and out all of the time. After I did some soul searching and worked through a lot of things, I saw things differently. Instead of looking for the changes externally, I started changing internally and that's when the attitude changed. My attitude about life is totally different now. I see the glass as half full instead of half empty. I live my life full of expectancy.

Wright

A lot of people are talking today about balancing their lives with families, homes, and careers. Balance is important to a healthy lifestyle. What advice can you give to people who have millions of things to do?

Moton

Balance is the key. My advice is not to overdo any ONE thing. Some things are good for us when done in moderation, but become bad for us when we overdo it. Yes, we have to work and work is good for us. But if you work too much, it can become bad. When you are working 10-12 hours days every day that means that you are neglecting other things you need to do. You are not getting your proper rest and when this happens you become susceptible to bad attitudes and diseases. Watching television can be relaxing, but watching too much of it can be bad because you are neglecting other things you need to do, including moving that body and getting more exercise. Playing and having a good time is good for you, but if you play too much it becomes bad because you are neglecting other duties. If you are doing any one thing too much—or doing too much period—it means that you are not taking care of yourself totally—mind, body, spirit and soul. Having a balanced lifestyle is important. Make sure that you have some downtime everyday. Many people say, "I don't have time to relax." Well, if you do not have at least 15-30 minutes everyday to relax, then you are TOO busy. We have to keep our lives in balance in order to be effective and productive people. Relaxation allows us to live whole, healthy and happy lives.

Wright

Joann, you juggle a full-time job, you have your own speaking and training business, you do a lot of acting, and you're an area Governor for Toastmasters International, and the beat goes on. How do you do it all?

Moton

I have to admit sometimes it becomes a little overwhelming. I'm learning how to focus on one thing at a time. I have a lot of things to juggle. When I think about everything at once that is when I become overwhelmed. So I try to make sure that I'm focusing on one thing at a time. Although I may have ten things to do in that day, I make sure I focus on the first thing first. Then I take the next one and the next one until I reach number ten. Focusing on each one, ONE at a time. I start my morning with prayer and meditation, scripture reading, exercises, and some laughter. This helps me to be focused for the day. I'm also learning how to say NO to some things, which sometimes can be a challenge for women because we try to do so much. But I have learned that it is better to say NO and do a few things well than to say yes to a lot of things and stress yourself out and do nothing well. So NO is a very important part of being able to juggle what I do. Try it sometime.

Wright

With juggling all these things, do you ever get stressed? If you do, what are some of the signs?

Moton

Oh yeah, there are times that I do get stressed and my body will let me know. My symptoms are, and I know them well, tightening of the shoulders, headaches, dry mouth, slurred and raspy voice, insomnia, forgetfulness and irritability. There was a time when I ran myself so much that I actually had an anxiety attack and I thought I was having a heart attack. That was enough for me to say that I have to slow down. Now I know the signs and I make sure that I key in on them and do something about them. Our bodies always give us signs and signals. Whether we pay attention to them or not. We can either pay attention to them or pay later. If we keep going our body is going to eventually shut down. I'm learning how to listen to my body. When I need rest, I take it. Sometimes that means grabbing five or ten minutes here or there to relax, not working through lunch—taking time away from my desk and taking a breather. You can take a stretch break. You can do some deep breathing exercises. Some of my favorite things to do to relax are to light a candle, sit in my favorite recliner, watch TV or read. I have a little fountain that has water that flows against rocks and that's very relaxing to me. Those are some of things that I do to relax. I also play with my two, three, and four-year old great-nephews and niece. They are lots of fun, so I play with them and that also helps me to de-stress.

Wright

How about laughter? How important is it to your well being?

Moton

I think it's really important. I encounter people everyday who appear to have a permanent frown on their faces. If they were to smile their face would crack. Humor is good for you. We cannot take life or ourselves too seriously. I use to be quite serious about everything. I still have my moments. All of my friends would tell me "You need to lighten up." Well, I am finally starting to take their advice. I can now laugh at myself (sometimes). You have to learn not to be too hard on yourself. Enjoy a funny movie or read a funny book. Laughter is a great de-stressor and it adds years to your life.

Wright

What about hobbies or recreational activities? How important are they to health and wellness?

Moton

People who just work all the time and don't have any type of recreational outlet or hobby have more stress. You need an outlet. You need a way to escape and get away from your regular routine, a way to rekindle your energy, rejuvenate and refocus. Hobbies can provide a way for you to get away from your routine. Do something that you thoroughly enjoy and immerse yourself in that. One of my hobbies is acting. I thoroughly enjoy that. I can become a totally different person and act totally different from my normal personality. I can escape the everyday routine by acting and doing different dramatic presentations; I enjoy doing that. I encourage people all the time to develop some type of positive outlet outside of work and their everyday routine; an outlet to avoid burnout.

Wright

I noticed an article in the State newspaper where you had done 40 Acres and a Prayer by Eugene Washington Productions. Is that a church sponsored thing? By the way, that Koger Center in Columbia, SC you performed in is really beautiful.

Moton

Yes, the Koger Center is awesome and it was a wonderful experience. Eugene Washington Productions sponsored the play. He wrote the play and performed in it as well. It was a tremendous experience. I played a role there that was totally, totally different from me. It was so much fun. I got to be a bad girl!

Wright

In researching for this interview something struck me in one of your Confidence Unlimited writings in one of the presentations you do called *Tapping Into the Power Within*. I'm going to quote you here. "No matter what obstacles you are faced with in life you have to believe that you can rise above it all. Even though you may have tried and failed many times you must believe that the next time you will succeed." That kind of goes along with something that you said, "Everyone is placed on earth for a purpose and that purpose is for each of us to make a positive difference in someone's life." So what do you do to help people get past the old mistakes and the life of failure that they've had, pick them back up and get them on the way to new challenges? What do you do through your company that helps that?

Moton

I tell people that they must face their fears and obstacles; admit that they exist and face them. Some people don't want to face the issues that have caused them to make mistakes. You have to find the root cause and then do whatever is needed to resolve the issues. There are many people, particularly African Americans, who do not believe in and do not seek counseling. They often say, "I don't need any counseling; I am not crazy," or "I am not paying anybody to listen to me." I do not agree. I am a big proponent of good counseling. I think it helps to have someone qualified and trained to help you dig through certain issues that you may have buried and forgotten were even there. These are the things that cause you to make the same mistakes over and over. A counselor can help you to get to the root of the problem, help you to address it, and to move forward. Another thing you must learn to do is to forgive. I am very much a living witness of the power of forgiveness. For many years I resented some things that my father had done; this affected my entire life. After I was able to forgive him, I began realizing my dreams, gifts and talents. When you are carrying around grudges, animosity and unforgiveness, you are weighed down with excess baggage. It's hard for you to move forward when you are burdened down with all that luggage. As Eryka Badu says, "Bag lady you are going to miss your bus carrying all that stuff." I encourage people to find the root cause of their problems. Figure out why you are making the mistakes you are making. It can be scary and painful, but it is worth it. It was painful for me, but just remember you are going *through* the pain. After you go through, you will then be able to really live a life filled with health and wellness. The key is to remember you are going through and you will come out on the other side. Trust me it works. I have done it. Everyone has the ability to live a successful, healthy and prosperous life. Everyone has that power within. Sometimes you have to go out and acquire some additional skills, but it's available to you. You just need to reach out and get it.

Wright

What great advice. It's really been a pleasure talking to you today, Joann. I want you to know that I appreciate you taking this much time with me for this interview. I think our readers are really going to learn a lot from your ideas and some of the things that you have been talking about today.

Moton

Thank you. It's been a pleasure talking to you, David.

Wright

Today we have been talking to Joann Moton. She is the President, Owner, and CEO of Confidence Unlimited and, as we have found out today, really knows a lot about healthy living, maintaining a balanced life, and getting on with life when you've been down before. Thank you so much, Joann, for being with us on *Conversations on Health and Wellness.*

About The Author

Joann Moton is the President and Owner and CEO of Confidence Unlimited, specializing in professional and personal development. The mission of the organization is to encourage, empower, and enable people to unleash their unlimited potential. Joann is an Advanced Toastmasters Gold and a District Officer of Toastmasters International.

Ms. Moton is a certified Professional Trainer and is available for seminars, workshops, training, and keynote addresses for businesses, schools, and other organizations on a local and national basis. Her services are designed to promote self-awareness and self-development. She is also an actress and uses her acting skills to present information in a dynamic, unique, interactive, and entertaining manner to increase retention and usage. The motto of her business is **"Confidence Unleashes the Potential of Unlimited Power."**

Joann Moton

Confidence Unlimited

P O Box 212478

Columbia, South Carolina 29221-2478

Phone: 803-731-2722 1

Phone: 1-866-LUV-SELF

Fax: 803-731-2722

Email: jmoton2005@aol.com

www.confidenceunlimited.com

Chapter 8

DR. EARL MINDELL

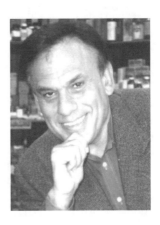

David E. Wright (Wright)

Today we are talking to Dr. Earl Mindell. Like Drs. Spock, Edell, and Ornish, Dr. Earl Mindell has become a household name to millions of North Americans. When the *Earl Mindell's Vitamin Bible* exceeded seven million worldwide, published in 30 languages, he had become a phenomenon. Currently it has sold over 10 million copies worldwide. Some of Dr. Mindell's previous books include, *Earl Mindell's Soy Miracle, Earl Mindell's Herb Bible,* and *Newer Bible Safe Eating, Food as Medicine, Shaping Up with Vitamins.* He conducts nutritional seminars around the world and makes daily appearances on radio and television programs. Dr. Mindell holds a Ph.D. in nutrition and is a professor of nutrition at Pacific Western University in Los Angeles. He is a California registered pharmacist and a master herbalist. He is a charter member of the American Academy of General Practice of Pharmacy as well as the American Pharmacist Association. Dr. Mindell, welcome to *Conversations on Health and Wellness.*

Dr. Earl Mindell (Mindell)

Well, it's a pleasure to be on the show. Actually I should add some of my other books too, *The Prescription Alternatives, The Diet Bible, The Allergy Bible*. I have got 47 books as of today and I'm working on a few more. I'm always working on more books.

Wright

I went to amazon.com just to check your book titles a few days ago.

Mindell

It's a little embarrassing. On amazon.com they have 95 things. They are not all, I mean some are tapes etc., but they've got almost everything. Some are out of print because I've been writing for 25 years now.

Wright

Dr. Mindell, millions of people are taking vitamin supplements today. However, in a recent article in *Biography Magazine*, you were quoted as saying, "Vitamins are no substitute for eating well." So, how do vitamins help the body?

Mindell

Well, let me say this. It's pathetic that the United States being one of the richest nations in the world, when it comes to nutrition, it's a third world country. So, vitamins don't replace a terrible diet, but you sure do need a supplementation because of this horrific diet that we're eating. I call it the "standard American dieter's fad." It's more like pathetic. I also call it the "Twinkie, Ding Dong, doughnuts, pizza, Prozac, Pepsi diet." So basically, vitamins work with food to produce energy. They are necessary for optimal health, which means your body is working as efficiently as possible, and for life as we know it. So it's important to get all the necessary nutrients. If you're lacking one vitamin, it can cause a problem with the other ones as well.

Wright

In the same article when asked about the secret to your success, you were quoted as saying, "I simply tell people the truth about how to take better care of themselves." From whom do people get erroneous information about their health?

Mindell

Well, they don't get any information about their health. They only get information about their sickness. I mean all you have to do is watch commercial television any particular night and you are inundated with all these drug ads for sickness. You don't hear anything about health. You know we call it health insurance, but it's not health insurance; it's sickness insurance. So we only hear about what to do in case you get sick. No one tells you about health or preventing, keeping this incredible body healthy. I mean we're living something like 77 years on the average doing what we do. I mean if we were to be really educated about how to take care of ourselves, 100 would be normal.

Wright

When the first edition of your book, *The Vitamin Bible*, came out in 1979, the medical community scorned you. You have said that, or they said that they thought you were a lunatic. In the past ten years, though, major research studies have changed, even the medical establishment's attitude. That must give you a tremendous satisfaction.

Mindell

Well, it does. In fact, last October in *The Journal of the American Medical Association,* they came out with a research article stating exactly that. That everyone should be taking a vitamin and mineral supplement. As I mentioned I'm an antique collector. I have quite a collection of antique pharmacy and medical things. I have a book from 1938 published by the American Medical Association. They were very big on vitamins! Of course, after the Second World War with the advent of the utilization of synthetic drugs like Penicillin, etc., the drug companies said, "Let's dump all of these old remedies and just concentrate on these synthetic drugs." And boy, they've done a pretty good job in the last 60 years. So it's not a new concept, but because the diet and the life style has changed so dramatically in this country, even the so-called establishment is becoming aware that there's no way you're going to get enough nutrients in your diet.

Wright

Last year, *The Journal of American Medical Association* reversed their 20 year old stance against vitamins.

Mindell

Correct.

Wright

What effect did that make on the public's attitude towards adding vitamins to their diet?

Mindell

Well, I think it definitely helps when you have the so-called establishment saying that it's imperative that people take a supplement. For instance, the March of Dimes, which is a pretty establishment charity, has ads going all over the place telling women of child bearing ages that they should be supplementing their diet with folic acid, one of the B vitamins. It prevents a birth defect called spina bifida, but it also does another thing too. A lack of folic acid, which just about everyone in the country has, causes the body to produce an over abundance of a toxic amino acid. Amino acids are the building blocks of protein called homocystine and that is probably a greater contributor to heart disease than elevated cholesterol. So by getting enough folic acid in the diet through supplementation, it will prevent this homocystine from being produced. You can see that we are learning that our diet is probably responsible for, I would say, 75 to 85% of the problems we have.

Wright

Dr. Mindell, you have said that low-fat diets have made people fatter than ever. How can that be?

Mindell

Well, that's a good question. You know we, a few years back—5 or 10 years back—we were told low-fat is the way to go and all of a sudden people started switching over to these low-fat or no-fat things. They didn't realize that these process food people would load them up with sugar and the processed carbohydrates. So it's pretty evident that no-fat or low-fat is not the way to go. I think we should decrease the amount of the processed carbohydrates and sugar. We're eating 150 pounds of sugar per person per year. To give you an idea how much sugar you're eating and don't even realize it, if you drink a typical 20 ounce soft drink, you're getting 14 teaspoons of sugar in that soft drink.

Wright

Wow! Goodness. I take a diet supplement every day that is time released. But the way I read your book, you almost have to take vitamins with food, do you not?

Mindell

Oh absolutely, you should be taking a vitamin supplement with food. I take a pack in the morning with breakfast and also with my evening meal. It's like, you know, you don't time release your food, so why should you time release the supplements? You should be taking them at least twice a day. Theoretically, you should take them three times a day, but that is very impractical for the average person. If I could get people to take them twice a day, I'd be happy.

Wright

And what they do is they supplement what you're not getting, right?

Mindell

They supplement what you're not getting and they make sure you're getting enough of what you should be getting.

Wright

Let me read a quote from you. "Each year 140 thousand Americans die from the adverse effects of prescription drug use and 938 thousand Americans are injured due to prescription and dispensing errors. Eleven million people are abusing prescription drugs. Drug companies are forming alliances with HMOs to control the drugs you take often at the expense of simpler, cheaper, and healthier lifestyle changes." Wow!

Mindell

Well, actually those statistics are a little bit out of date. It's about 140 Americans die from prescription drug use outside of hospitals and another 100 thousand in hospitals. So, if you really were to take the amount of people in the United States dying from prescription drugs, it's probably the fourth leading cause of death.

Wright

Wow!

Mindell

It's getting worse. Let me tell you something. We are definitely subsidizing the world when it comes to the cost of drugs. We pay more than anywhere else in the world. People are getting prescriptions filled in Canada at half the price as the United States.

Wright

So how do we reverse this trend?

Mindell

Well, we start promoting wellness. You know, if you're well, you don't need prescription drugs. What a fantastic idea that is! I mean we have our politicians running around the country saying we have to cut the price of prescription drugs for the elderly and they go on to generic drugs. Well if they are healthy, they don't need prescription drugs.

Wright

Dr. Mindell, it would seem that with all the research about the importance of good health, we are in a revolution. Where do you see the future of the wellness revolution?

Mindell

I see something that was talked about in the book that said, and I agree, that the wellness business, if you want to call it that, is going to become bigger than the sickness business. It will be a one trillion-dollar business because people are living longer. They want a better quality of life and they want to be in good shape in the last years of their life. I mean big deal you live an extra year or two years longer if you're put away in a convalescent hospital or connected to some machine. That not what you want. So we're better educated. We're much more informed of this whole thing. And this is a wellness revolution. It's too expensive to continue what we've done before, and that's wait until you get sick and try to pay to get well.

Wright

You know, I was looking at one of the articles that you were one of the contributors to in a magazine. It had listed several vitamins starting at A and going through B1, B6, and D and C and all. I just started reading what these things do for you. Vitamin A, for example, the benefits if I read correctly here are essential to eye health, builds resistance to respiratory infections.

Mindell

Right.

Wright

It boosts the immune system, promotes strong bones, healthy skin, hair teeth and gums.

Mindell

Right.

Wright

So why in the world?

Mindell

Well, you know, you said we're probably contemporaries when it comes to age. I remember when I was a little boy, I grew up in western Canada, a very cold climate, and in the winter my mother would give us a spoon of fish liver oil. I think we would run to school faster because it tasted so horrible, of course, fish liver oil is a good source of vitamin A and D. You know, in a cold climate, you're not outside very much and you don't get the sun, so vitamin D was important. Vitamin A is an anti-infective vitamin, and yet we know nothing now. Today we don't give our children fish oil. We give them antibiotics. So maybe they knew something back then that we have kind of ignored.

Wright

Let's change the subject for just a minute. What do you think of the Surgeon General's report on obesity in the United States?

Mindell

It's about time! I'm glad that they finally came out, the Surgeon General came out and now calls obesity and over weight a disease state. Actually it was the last Surgeon General. He has stated that 300 thousand Americans die every year from the complications of obesity such as heart disease, such as diabetes, such as hardening of the arteries, high blood pressure, strokes, and how about this one? If we could get people's weight back to normalcy because we're not, two out of three Americans are over weight, well if the average American was at an average normal weight, 40% of the cancers that we are afflicted with would not occur. Forty. 4-0. It's about time. In fact, yesterday in one of the national newspapers' headlines, one third of Americans born in 2000 will get diabetes, and that's pretty frightening to think that we're bringing up a generation where a third of the children are going to be diabetic.

Wright

Goodness. You know, as I looked at all the information about vitamins, I ran across the definition of minerals. Now, do you mix the two or are they mutually exclusive or what. For example, I was interested in this one, I guess it's called selenium because I'm 64 and it acts as an anti-oxidant, which I really don't understand. It says it slows the aging process.

Mindell

Well, let me say this. I really should have called my book *The Vitamin Mineral Bible*, but minerals are kind of like the Cinderella of the nutrition world. They don't get the play that vitamins do, but they are as important, if not more important, than vitamins. You can not make a single mineral in your body, so the two, of course, work together. But the main thing to mention about selenium is that it is not only antioxidant, but it also has anti-cancer properties, and it's found in things that people don't eat—onions, garlic, brown rice, and seafood. It works along with vitamin E and other anti-oxidants to make it even more potent. But as an oxidant, okay, here's the best way to describe what it does. There's the good guys and the bad guys. The good guys are called antioxidants, and the bad guys are called radical oxygen molecules that are caused to increase by stress, by your so-called the things in diets that are called the fat cats, fat, alcohol, tobacco, sugar, and salt. They increase the radical oxygen molecules from being produced. The bad guys speed up the aging process and lead to degenerative diseases, like heart disease, cancer, and stroke, etc. We're not dying of old age. We're dying of degenerative diseases, which I feel that 80 or 85% can be prevented. But you want to have more of the good guys in your body than the bad guys. Selenium, vitamin E, the carotenoids, vitamin C, things such as green tea and grape seed, soy foods and garlic are a very rich source of antioxidants. All these foods and nutrients help to neutralize the bad guys. Isn't it pathetic though. You know here's yourself, I'm sure a well educated person who knows so little about these health issues, but I'll bet you, you know which drug to have if you have a headache.

Wright

You know it's embarrassing. I've spent half my life in some school or another, but my gosh, it's unbelievable how little I know.

Mindell

There is such a need to really reeducate people about wellness. I think it's going to happen only because of the financial situation. Once people start being really hit in their pocketbook, I mean, anybody who has so-called sickness insurance knows every year it keeps going up and up and up and there's no end to it. If you haven't had a prescription filled recently, the average prescription now is $65.00 on the way to $100.00. You say, "Oh I have a policy that I pay a co-payment." Well, watch out because that co-payment is going to be close to $25.00 to $50.00 very soon.

Wright

Right, and actually medical insurance in this country now we don't take out medical insurance. We just make monthly payments on our medical bill.

Mindell

Exactly.

Wright

Even though you pay just a small portion of the co-pay, the other is indicated in your premium.

Mindell

Then there's the thing called taxes, too. You might have heard of those. So if we continue to do this, if we don't start focusing on wellness and prevention, we're going to bankrupt the country.

Wright

With our book, *Conversations on Health and Wellness*, we're trying to encourage our readers to be better, to live better, and be more fulfilled by listening to the examples of our guest authors. Is there anything or anyone in your life that has made a difference for you and helped you to become a better person?

Mindell

Well, absolutely. My mentors are many. I knew Linus <u>Pauling,</u> an amazing, brilliant scientist who was into this all on vitamin C, etc., Jack La Lane has always been one of my heroes. Still in his upper 80's, has been exercising forever. He says he still doesn't like to exercise but he does it anyway. I can go back to Robert Cummings, an actor that was into this in the '20s, and I had the opportunity to meet the Shute brothers from London, Ontario, who were the first people who did the research on vitamin E. It goes on and on, but I think the big thing that I'd really try to tell people is that we have got to take as good care of ourselves as we do our dogs, cats, automobiles, and rose bushes. If you really look at it, most people take better care of their cars than they do themselves. I mean, you hear these ads all the time. Every 3,000 miles take your car in for changing oil, and make sure this is in order, and people get their car washed on a regular basis. Well, how about our bodies, why don't we know how to take care of them? I think when a baby is born it should have a maintenance manual. That probably would be a good idea.

Wright

Robert Cummings, boy I tell you, that brings back great memories.

Mindell

He was a wonderful man.

Wright

He was young looking.

Mindell

He was young looking. He was into this back in the '20s. I had an opportunity of knowing him and learning from him. This field is not new; it probably started in the '20s. When we found them, we've learned so much and we're doubling our knowledge or our nutrition every 18 months. Yet the average person is still in the dark, doesn't hear anything about this, and they really should.

Wright

I remember, oh 25, 30, 35 years ago, I got involved in this company called Nutri-Bio that was some vitamin company, and Cummings was one of the ....

Mindell

He was the spokesperson for that company.

Wright

Yeah, and I'll tell you, he was taking vitamins daily. I mean morning, noon, and night.

Mindell

Well, guess what? I still am and I'm 63 now; I've been doing this for 40 years. I'll tell you I get compliments all the time by people saying, "Yeah, you look 15, 20 years younger than you are."

Wright

If you could have a platform, Dr. Mindell, and tell our readers something that you feel would help them or encourage them, what would you say?

Mindell

I would say that if you want to be healthy, you have got to take the responsibility of your health in your own hands. It's as simple as that. If you want to be sick, don't worry about a thing. It's going to happen. They are waiting for you at $3,000.00 a day. They have got a nice hospital bed. They are ready to come with the paramedics in the ambulance to pick you up.

Wright

Today we have been talking to Dr. Earl Mindell, who has become a household name in the health and wellness industry. And as we have found out today, probably knows as much if not more about vitamins and minerals than any man that lives on this planet. Dr. Mindell, I really appreciate the time you have spent with me today.

Mindell

Thank you and stay healthy.

About The Author

Dr. Earl Mindell, worldwide best-selling author of the *Vitamin Bible* and dozens of other books, has taught countless people all he knows about health and nutrition. Through the use of herbs and vitamins, Dr. Mindell's exclusive nutrition formulations have helped perhaps millions of people lose weight, look younger and feel better.

Dr. Earl Mindell
Phone: 1-888-345-6709
www.drearlmindell.com

Chapter 9

Debra Novotny, L.Ac; D. Hom; ND

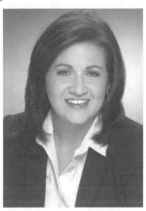

THE INTERVIEW

David E. Wright (Wright)

What if you had the rare opportunity from an early age to study with great minds about ancient, natural forms of health care? Debra Novotny had such an opportunity. She began her studies of meditation, fitness, healing, and natural healing at the age of fourteen. A mentor in her life introduced her to the art of healing from the Middle East (India) and Far East (Asian) through a variety of teachers. This region was the main home for most of man-kind five-thousand plus years ago. Her studies lead to looking for answers on how to heal yourself and stay well naturally. She coupled her strong belief in God or a higher power with the fact that in all spiritual writings mankind spoke of natural healing tools and plants. This was just the beginning.

Today, Debra is an alternative health care physician, author and public speaker. She has a dynamic Health & Wellness practice in Denver, Colorado. She is licensed in Oriental Medicine and holds certifications in many other fields of alternative medicine. Her natural, alternative medicine approaches include acupuncture, Oriental medicine, homeopathy, herbs, and yoga. She blends ancient science with

21st century cutting edge medicine in her custom-designed Enhanced Living Today programs, internet magazine, teleclasses and products.

She is a member of the National Certification Commission for Acupuncture and Oriental Medicine (NCCAOM) and American Association of Naturopathic Physicians (AANP). Debra, welcome to *Conversations on Health and Wellness.*

Debra Novotny (Novotny)
Thank you, David. I'm excited to be here.

Wright
Unlike many speakers, you juggle an alternative health care practice, teleclasses, workshops and on line programs to help people with health and wellness. You've been quoted as stating your mission is to bring health and wellness to individual people around the world. How did you start on such a mission?

Novotny
David, I occasionally ask myself that question. The answer that comes to mind for me is that Healing is Spiritual. This was the first lesson I learned from my first teacher. There really is a mind, body, soul connection. Starting out, my goal was to take the knowledge I had learned and help people feel better, and simply come home every night to my own family.

Soon I realized that I was on a personal mission to do something not done before. My undying thirst for knowledge and the desire to help others and myself experience wellness, not illness, continued to propel me into reaching out to more teachers and mentors. Since my own health was poor, I believed I was looking for personal safety and a cure. Perhaps I was. I am one of those rare people where my hobby became my occupation. I am blessed that I do what I love and love what I do.

Wright
I know many of our readers will be most interested in learning your definition of alternative health and wellness?

Novotny
David, alternative health and wellness is everything other than standard western health care. That means acupuncture, homeopathy, and Oriental medicine, Ayurvedic or Vedic Medicine. It also includes

natural medicine where we use nutrition, both American and Chinese herbs, yoga, tai chi, massage, and any form of Energetic Medicine like Chakras and intuitive medicine. But it's not limited to just these main areas. Essential oils is also a tool of alternative medicine. Western medicine includes western drugs, surgery, Physical Therapy, and some types of spinal adjustment care. We work closely with some chiropractors that still practice natural or straight chiropractic.

Wright

You talk a lot about a mind, body, and soul connection. What do you mean by this?

Novotny

Alternative medicine works on five levels of a person. Physical, emotional, mental, body chemistry, and energetic. There are seven energies that are involved in wellness according to many of the ancient seers, especially those of India. It's not simply performing acupuncture or eating right. You have to consciously be treated and begin healing on all these levels. The practitioner has to know *how to work at each level*. Acupuncture for instance, is a tool for the practitioner or physician of acupuncture. Unless they have training also in Ancient East Indian (India) Energetic work on the meridians, Chakras, and a person's energy field they will not reach the core of the problem. In my opinion, one must also study the medicine of India to heal the energy of the meridians of Oriental medicine and visa versa.

I say this only because we can trace the beginnings back to India from Asia, Babylon, Egypt, Ireland, and Greece. These are usually the realms of ancient history. Where we find the tapestry of history we find the tools of alternative or natural healing, the key to Wellness.

Wright

Is this different than say healing touch, Reki or something like that?

Novotny

Yes it is. These are modern forms of Chinese Qi Gong work. Qi Gong is part of Oriental medicine. Unfortunately very few acupuncturists incorporate it into their treatments. Qi Gong takes years to learn and full understanding of Oriental Medicine and acupuncture are needed.

Wright

Where do things like herbs, homeopathy, and nutrition come in?

Novotny

With herbs they must be of the highest quality. The source is everything. Then you have to know how they are prepared. The mixture is vital as it releases a synergistic affect on the healing of the body both physically and energetically. The problem is high quality prescription herbs are only sold through Alternative Health Physicians. We're working on making some of these available to clients on line without a prescription. When you purchase from a health food store you're buying your health from a sales clerk. I don't care what weekend nutrition class they took. Herbs are medicine.

Homeopathy is pure energy medicine. But you know the remarkable thing about it is that it works on the physical body too. Some people may not know what homeopathy is. It is a plant or substance that is diluted and percussed to make a tincture that has no side-effects.

It is safe for children and the aged. I do not recommend taking it though without guidance. It is medicine. This means instead of side-effects you may experience a healing reaction and not know what to do. With a trained homeopath you have a coach that can first make sure you take the best potency for you. This will reduce the possibility of a healing reaction greatly. If you still have a healing reaction a homeopath will be able to help you.

My homeopathic background is in using single remedy and multi-remedy homeopathics. I also use Essential Chinese Oils and these are stellar in their ability to work on all levels of healing. There is only one source that I know of that makes real Chinese Essential Oils.

An example of how wonderful these oils are is I recently used a formula on a client for anxiety and stress. She had tightness in her chest with shortness of breath, insomnia, dizziness, and fullness in her head. I placed one drop on her palm and she rubbed them together and then over her upper chest. By the next day all her symptoms were gone and she has been fine since.

Nutritional supplementation should only be done with someone who knows how to work with nutrition. I have had people bring in 15 different bottles of stuff and they didn't need any of it. Even the multi-vitamin they had picked up somewhere was causing them problems. Another client was having terrible gas and bloating mid-day. I tried everything. Finally one day she brought in a bag full of stuff. I had asked her many times if she was taking anything other than what I had put her on and she always said no. It was the multi-vitamin. She had thought I meant other things like drugs or something another health providers had given her. She didn't think that what she bought at the store herself was medicine. We got her on the right vitamin and the gas and bloating are gone.

Wright

How do you do this if you are working with a client "remotely" meaning someone who never comes into your practice?

Novotny

As a medical Intuitive, I work with other tools as well. These are simple things like intuition and understanding a person's health problems and their wellness goals. In India there is also another tool called Jyotish. My intuition coupled with Jyotish, which could be referred to as the science of using the energy fields of all that is around the client, allows me to map out so-to-speak what is happening at that moment for the client and approach not only their health and wellness but other aspects of their life if we desire to. Jyotish is something I also utilize with my patients if they wish.

Wright

How long have these Energetic health approaches been around?

Novotny

Oriental medicine is about 3,000 to 5,000 years old, but India has records of using Energetic medicine since 8,000 BCE. Greece, Egypt, and Asia brought out or borrowed parts of India's Vedic system of Wellness. In fact, every form of medicine that is natural uses energy to some level. The biggest fear factor I have about western drugs is that they block the body's natural flow of energy.

Wright

Sounds like knowing how to work with a person's energy is important regardless of if you are doing acupuncture or some other form of health care?

Novotny

It's the single biggest reason most people don't heal and experience wellness. Other factors that are important are movement in your life if you don't like to exercise, do yoga or Tai Chi. These are recommended even if you bike, run, or lift weights. This can add over 10 years of *healthy living* if you just do yoga or Tai Chi 3-4 times a week.

Eating well for your health can add 10 or 20 more years of *healthy living* to your life.

"Mind your mind." Your thoughts and words are very powerful. Listen to your self talk. Are you telling yourself that you hurt? That you are old? If you are doing this we have resources for you. This alone can keep you from being as well as you can be.

As I said before, work with someone who really understands working with *your* energetic-self. That means someone well versed in meridians, Chakras, aura or energy body, Vedic and Oriental medicine. A high understanding of herbal medicine and Homeopathy is also important as these are also energetic in nature.

This medicine reaches all levels of a person; physical, mental, emotional and energetic.

Wright

I can see how that would be important. I mean there are people who have a physical injury but also suffer from an emotional component as well right?

Novotny

Yes, take a person who has irritable bowel for instance. They have stomach pain, bloating, constipation and diarrhea, and other physical symptoms that bring them to seek alternative health care like acupuncture and herbal/homeopathic medicine.

Often they suffer from worry and stress. The may be feel ungrounded also. Now let's look at just these 3 additional symptoms. Worry is an emotion. Stress is a mental trait and the ungrounded feeling is energetic.

Drugs or surgery are not the answer for *any* of these symptoms. The IBS or irritable bowel will respond wonderful to acupuncture and treatment with correcting the nutrition, adding to the diet nourishing and supportive herbs, homeopathics, and nutritional care.

For the worry and stress we may want to add Qi Gong, Yoga, or Tai Chi to relax the body and the mind. Meditation works wonders as well.

For emotions and mental disharmony, I also use massage, essential Chinese oils mixed in the lotion that we use and I use Intuitive medicine to move the energy in the body.

My clients and patients actually feel the movement and balancing of energy in their body as I work. This isn't healing touch. Its true ancient Energy work from the Middle East, Far East and India, which I consider kind of in-between, but that is a history lesson for another time.

Wright

I want to make sure we touch on the fact that you have a virtual wellness program and what that means. After all, our readers are looking for answers to health problems and that is what you do isn't it?

Novotny

Absolutely. Our goal is to solve health problems, help clients stop making health mistakes, stay young, and enjoy wellness. There are ways to do this no matter what age you start at or what state your health is in.

Wright

How do you do this virtually?

Novotny

We have a number of websites that allow the client or patient to find the right program or personal plan for them. Some people live in the Denver area and they become patients, but for those that don't we also offer ways to invest in their personal health and wellness via the internet, telephone clinics or workshops, and conferences I host all over the world.

Wright

Learning all this must have taken a long time. I mean you are known for blending together Ancient Medicine from many different cultures with 21st century Quantum Medicine.

Novotny

I always ask the client to imagine, "How much this is worth to you?" Whether they come to see me or begin to work with me by internet or phone. I make a point to meet every client personally even if it's by phone. But back to your question . . .

I started studying over thirty years ago. Let's do the math in real dollars and time spent if a person were to do what I have done to learn all this and create a unique one of a kind program. This program any one can simply do regardless of where they live through our virtual system.

Every year since I was 14 years old I made sure I studied with a master somewhere, and have done so for 10 of every 12 months each year. In today's dollars it would cost almost $816,000.00 for this much education and experience. I have studied with at least 35 mentors and teachers from around the globe.

My teachers and mentors come from Western Medicine, Middle Eastern Medicine, Far Eastern Medicine, Native American Medicine, South American Medicine, German Homeopathic Medicine, Greek Medicine, and many ancient and modern medical sciences.

So when I see a patient or client they're getting the expertise of over 35 of the top Alternative health and wellness experts and the savings of hundreds of thousands of dollars. This doesn't even take into account the amount of time I have devoted to this work. Plus, they get me and I am a master of what I do.

I almost forgot to mention that this work I have blended together dates back to 10,000 BCE. Bringing together millions of health and wellness masters and experts.

Wright

What a value this is to your clients and patients. Can you share with us in-depth the path you took to learn all this?

Novotny

It's actually fun to learn I guess if you are me. I sometimes think how I could spend my time and money on something else, but I really love my work and this is an investment of time and money to help others. That's really rewarding to me.

I began studying yoga exercise and meditation. I found it was the only thing that stopped my migraines. Later in life, I quite doing it and my migraines returned so I personally know the value of yoga. It also helped my allergies and bronchitis. I went to yoga five nights a week and once a month I would travel 100 miles to work with a swami and study. I was only 14 at the time. My teacher drove me to study with the swami—her master teacher. Together, they taught me about the medicine of India and the Vedas. This of course added other mentors in Middle Eastern medicine and science. The financial cost at the time is nothing compared to the classes I attend now. One of my current mentors charges $10,000 per weekend to study with him.

I help people who can't afford to work with him and my work is much different. We each have a destiny; mine is to help a certain niche of people that can't afford this level of Wellness care, but need it none the less. My clients are people just like you and me.

Everyone who becomes a client or patient and follows their personal treatment plan gives me a testimonial to the positive changes in their health and wellness. Many comment on how we work to help blend their new wellness into their lives and the positive changes that happen not only to their health but their relationships, wealth, spiritual path, success and much more.

Since my work blends what I have learned from many mentors not just a few, there is no other personalized program available like what I do and there never will be.

Each client's health problem is individual and I create an individual wellness plan for them.

Wright

Can you tell us more about your internet websites and the services?

Novotny

We have 2 main websites to choose from:

www.alternativehealthmentor.com
www.enhancedlivingtoday.com

The Alternative Health Mentor offers you an array of health problem solving tools and tips. We offer the book series Ancient Remedies. A few of our titles are: The 5 Secrets to Stopping the Cold & Flu; 21 Days to NO Allergies; The 14 Biggest Mistakes Arthritis Suffers Make; 5 Ways to Stay Young; The Lose Weight Without Dieting Handbook; Let Go of Back Pain; Cure Carpel Tunnel <u>Without</u> Drugs or Surgery; and many more.

Wright

I hear you mentor clients from around the world. How do you do that?

Novotny

One way is through www.alternativehealthmentor.com. A client can take tele-clinics, tele-workshops and attend seminars or conference in their own city or town.

Wright

How do the telephone clinics and workshops work?

Novotny

You can see the upcoming topics and events on our events calendar at www.alternativehealthmentor.com. Each month I host at least 2 tele-phone programs. The programs hold up to 50 or more callers. Often they fill up so we tell people to phone in about 5 minutes early to be sure to make the call.

The caller simply has to sign-up on our website for the class they want and we email them the phone number to call and the time of the clinic. When they call in we have a wonderful interactive program that you can listen to right from your home or office.

If they can't make a call, we tape all classes and they can listen to them by downloading the CD, or read them by downloading the manuscript. Some of our classes are free and others our fee-based.

The topic of our classes change every month. They may be on allergies such as 10 Ways *You Can Stop Insomnia WITHOUT Drugs*. And we may also offer that month a 2-part clinic titled *Simple Steps to Stopping Irritable Bowel*.

If you miss a health problem we usually have it available on CD or in a manuscript of the call.

Wright

How do you know what people want to know about?

Novotny

Each month on this website we *ask* them to tell us what they want to know about. When you go to this site you will see an "AskDrDebra" box where you can ask me your most burning question on a health problem.

Wright

That's amazing! You ask the public what they want to know about the most regarding a health problem and then you have a tele-class to answer their questions and solve their problems?

Novotny

That's it. We offer what the public asks for and we help them avoid the most common mistakes they may be making. We provide ways to better health, solving their health issue, and enjoying wellness in their lives.

Wright

What about your acclaimed newsletter, *Alternative Health Reporter?*

Novotny

From this same site you can join the *Alternative Health Reporter.* It's free and offers tips for a health problem each month, and highlights another area of your life so you can enjoy the "Enhanced Living™" experience. It also contains another "AskDrDebra" box for a different health problem.

Wright

Enhanced Living Today™? Isn't that your self-development plan that helps people tie all the areas of their life together?

Novotny

Yes, and our website is www.enhancedlivingtoday.com. We offer a free E-course that ties the 7 areas of life together so that you can truly have the "Life You Desire." Enhanced Living *Today* takes you a step further than just changing your health. Our clients that want to enhance every facet of their lives find this site more in-depth. Think about it David, health is connected to how you're doing in your relationships, your finances, and how you feel about yourself?

If you save and save for retirement only to find that you neglected your health along the way how do you end up spending your retirement money? On health problems and you become stressed. That affects your relationships. How successful do you feel at this point?

Wright

Does this get very involved? Most people don't want something that takes a long time.

Novotny

We're back to the beginning. I have already done all the research and studying. I have spent the time and the huge expense the client doesn't have to.

One thing I noticed when learning all this; each conference, seminar, workshop, and teacher showed me a piece or one thing, but I had to study for over 30 years to get all the pieces.

What I do is create a personal health problem solving plan so the client doesn't have to learn all this, take years to do so or spend a fortune to do so.

Let me ask this one…But how much is all this worth? It's worth a lot more than I charge. I had one lady send me a tip after she completed her plan saying I should charge more and that what she got was worth thousands. Of course I sent the check back with a thank you for such a wonderful compliment.

The plain answer in solving your health problem *is* easy and fast. It's not like taking a pill though where you hide the problem but you feel better for a few hours. Real wellness lasts days, weeks and into months and years. It won't happen over night and it takes your personal desire to be well. I will mentor you and help you, but you live with yourself daily. You can't be a bystander in your own life.

Wright

Your other two sites how can the reader benefit from them?

Novotny

Our internet sites are always growing and changing so look at each regularly. We also have two other minor websites. The www.askdebranovotny.com internet website is a free standing "Ask-DrDebra" site that we gather an array of answers to questions that affect everyday life and living. www.alternativehealthportal.com is a just that a portal where you can find other information, services, and products most not connected with me or my work. I realize that I don't have all the answers and I want to offer a more targeted "search engine" if you will for the public.

Wright

Sounds like there are many different way to obtain wellness?

Novotny

Definitely. Even within my health and wellness plans they must be customized to some degree for the individual client.

Wright

Your approach to wellness is very different. I've heard that most alternative practitioners use just one thing and they have gone the western approach of treating the same illness the same way in all their clients instead of looking at the person. How do you feel about this?

Novotny

It did happen to some but there are many great healers out there. We work with alternative healers all over the world. Part of our online plan is that you have someone local to treat you. Often our clients come to us with their wellness investment team already in place and add us to it.

Remember we talked about planning for retirement? How many people plan for Wellness? Not many. The few that do live longer stay younger and their golden years are healthy ones where they enjoy their retirement.

Those that don't plan usually end up sick and unable to do the things they planned. One of the first things you'll learn working with me in my office or on-line is to plan your wellness. Invest in a wellness team. Select one or up to three wellness experts to assist with wellness. I hope I am one of the people you select and you should have an acupuncturist, massage therapist and may be one other healer depending on your current health issues. If your acupuncturist doesn't also have expertise in herbs, homeopathy, Chinese Essential Oils and nutrition, this would be the person you want to add or perhaps a traditional or what is called a straight chiropractor.

Wellness care lasts a life time so don't expect to regain your health and then move on. You don't contribute to a retirement plan for a few months and expect to have anything when you retire so don't treat your own health with less investment.

Once your health issues are solved you can usually enjoy visiting your massage therapist and acupuncturist once or twice a month. Many of my patients come in every two months unless something happens and then we take care of the health problem and get them back out enjoying their lives.

Wright

You also do speaking for companies, associations, conferences locally and across the country. How do our readers book you?

Novotny

Call me. We have a toll-free number 866-332-7266. I am a member of the Doctor's Speakers Bureau and our non-profit organization's goal is to educate people. You can look on the site to see some of the topics I speak on or phone my office.

Wright

Why is so important to make sure your alternative health care physician has certain training in various fields?

Novotny

If you don't you could spend valuable time in treatment that isn't right for you. Make sure they know what they are doing and that they have certification to back it up. Check how long they have practiced each field and don't go to someone who you don't feel right about.

If the physician is trained at a true Oriental Medicine school they will have gone through at least 6 or more years of schooling and be a member of the NCCAOM. This is very important as it means they went to an accredited school not a weekend program offered through the AMA or the chiropractic association. That's a big requirement we can talk about later.

I use this example. Would you take your baby to the doctor that delivered them or to a pedestrian? Or you can think of it this way. What if you owned a Porsche and a Honda? Would you take the Porsche to the Honda dealer for repairs? Your health is your most valued asset.

Wright

In closing what is the single most important step one can take toward wellness?

Novotny

Starting today on a wellness program and working with a mentor to stay on target. Don't waste your health. If you knew you could live to be 120 years old and have great health would you like to?

Your body and your mind are made to live that long. Take wellness into your life and live long and healthy.

Wright

Today we have been talking to Debra Novotny. Thank you Debra for being with us today on *Conversations on Health and Wellness*.

About The Author

Debra Novotny has devoted 34 years to the study and practice of health, wellness, and *Enhanced Living Today™*

Debra's has a wellness practice, mentors clients world-wide and has internet based programs for all her clients. She helps you blend the 7 areas of your life together and live the life you truly desire.

Each *Enhanced Living Today™* program is personalized for you or your business. Debra is available to speak at your workshop, seminar, associations, conference, and other venues.

Debra holds degrees in Oriental Medicine, Homeopathy, and Natural Medicine. She also is known as a premiere Intuitive and Spiritual healer.

Debra Novotny, L.Ac; D. Hom; ND

Accent On Health

5924 So. Kipling Pkwy. Suite N

Littleton, Colorado 80127

Phone: 303-989-2727

Phone: 866-332-7266

Email: debra@enhancedlivingtoday.com

www.alternativehealthmentor.com

www.enhancedlivingtoday.com

Chapter 10

WENDY KAUFMAN

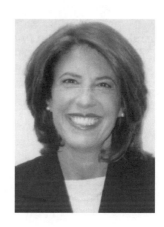

THE INTERVIEW

David E. Wright (Wright)

Wendy Kaufman was born and raised in Westchester, New York. She earned a Bachelor's Degree in Education from Syracuse University and went on to complete her Master's Degree in Industrial Psychology at the University of Pennsylvania. Following graduation she joined the human resources division at the Hertz Corporation, where she concentrated on compensation issues. From Hertz, Wendy made a career transition when she joined Fordham University where she held various positions and moved on to Yeshiva University where she was the Director of Career Placement. After leaving Yeshiva, she spent several years working as a consultant before finally taking the plunge and forming her own company, Balancing Life's Issues, Inc. (BLI). The company specializes in motivational programs, keynote speaking and professional training sessions. Among the many companies BLI, Inc. has proudly served are: IBM; J.P. Morgan; Chase; Johnson & Johnson; *The New York Times;* and Coach. With a rebooking rate of 100%, Wendy and her stellar group of trainers plan to continue BLI 's growth and success by continuing to motivate, inspire and train America's workforce. Wendy Kaufman, welcome to *Conversations on Health and Wellness.*

Wendy Kaufman (Kaufman)

Thank you.

Wright

Tell me when you first started public speaking.

Kaufman

I started public speaking when I was in the school band in fourth grade. The problem with my being in the band was that I could not play an instrument. However, instead of kicking me out of the program, our brilliant band director asked me to be the announcer for the band. Even at that age I really enjoyed speaking to an audience. I was hooked and that was the beginning of my public speaking career.

Wright

I've been booking speakers for the last 14 years and I always ask them this question. What makes you different as a public speaker?

Kaufman

There are so many great speakers and each one brings their own unique voice to the work. One of the things that sets me apart is the fact that I'm a single mom with three kids and I run a busy, successful company and I use all of it to inform my speaking. I'm very candid and honest about the very personal trials and tribulations of my life. Audiences can immediately relate to me on many different levels, which is very rewarding. People really appreciate hearing the good, the bad, and the ugly about my life because most of them can find similarities to their own lives. It makes my speeches very personal and I think I earn the trust of my audiences because I'm willing to reveal the truth of my own life. It's very difficult to put yourself and your life on the line but it makes such an impact on my audiences and the work that I'm willing to do it.

Wright

So what is your message?

Kaufman

My message is that it is imperative for all of us to learn to balance our lives and the new issues that we're continually confronted with. When I was in graduate school, I did my dissertation on something called Dual Career Relationships. At that time many of my professors thought I was barking up the wrong tree—they didn't believe that dual career relationships and the problems that would be implied within such relationships would ever become an important issue. They just didn't see it happening. They believed that the traditional family dynamic would prevail. Well, how many years later and we learn that the traditional family only makes up 20% of American households today. So here we are in uncharted territory. How do we function in this new paradigm and balance work and family? It's the number two issue concerning corporate America. The number one issue is communication, which of course plays right into the ability to balance. So here we have two brand new skills that really need to be taught just like computer training and accounting. We need to learn how to balance our work and our family and we need to learn how to communicate with them as well.

Wright

Tell me more about your laughter therapy.

Kaufman

That's one of my favorite classes! Charlie Chaplin coined a phrase back in the 20's, "Take the pain and play with it." Laughter and finding humor in situations is nothing new, but learning how to use it, especially in the workplace is a fairly new concept. Many celebrities have used the idea of laughing at themselves to create very successful careers and TV shows. Just look at Jerry Seinfeld, Roseanne and Ray Romano. However, most of us don't really think of humor and laughter as being all that important in our lives. Do you know that an average four year old laughs 400 times a day? They don't think about whether it's a Monday or a Saturday—they have fun just because it's a new day. When I ask people if they are having fun at work the most common answer I get is something like, "No, it's a Monday, it's a work day. It's not the right time for fun. " We spend most of our waking time at work—much more time than we spend at home and with our families. If we decide that we can't have fun when we are working, that doesn't leave us much time when we're not working, does it? Medical research has proved that laughter truly is the best medicine. It has been shown to boost the immune system, alleviate depression and because laughing releases beta endorphins, it simply makes us feel better.

Wright

I can see Balancing Life's Issues as a title for a keynote, but you named your company Balancing Life's Issues. Where did that come from?

Kaufman

I am interested in exploring both the positive and negative impact of life's issues and in finding the balance in between. After September 11 we were all faced with an unprecedented set of new issues and trauma, especially here in New York. After the initial shock wore off a lot of us wondered how we would ever get back on our feet again—how could we possibly move on following such a terrible and terrifying event? Well, it was about learning to recognize all of these issues, some new, like terrorism, some old like our families, children, the environment, aging parents, money and balancing them with all of the requirements of our lives. One of my most popular speeches is about living on your paycheck, and getting out of debt. Debt is a crisis facing millions of Americans today. The notion that money can buy happiness gets us into a lot of trouble. We'll buy something because we get that shopper's high, and then we're pretty happy for about 20 minutes, or until we get the bill and realize that we are living in debt. I suggest that there are many other ways to make yourself and your family happy that don't cost anything. I ask audiences to think of things that they enjoy doing that are free, like cooking with the family. This is an invaluable tool that not only saves money, but creates closeness within your family. I use myself as an example. After my divorce, which was anything but amicable, I was broke and had to come up with new routes to happiness for me and for my kids. It was tough, but I discovered a million things that we can do together without breaking the bank and spending a millions dollars.

Wright

What are some of the most poignant stories that you have, perhaps from various speeches that you've given?

Kaufman

I often talk about my health when I was in the process of getting divorced. I was under a tremendous amount of stress and for the most part I felt ok, just stressed. I started to have terrible problems with my teeth and gums and finally went to the doctor only to find out that my stress and anxiety were manifesting in my mouth. People respond to this story by writing to tell me that they had been experiencing problems with their eyes, their arms, one person wrote and told me that he thought he was having a heart attack, but didn't want to tell anyone—he thought it was just stress and didn't realize what a serious impact it can have on the body. After hearing my story these people finally sought some kind of help and averted even more serious problems. It's so powerful and moving—that by sharing my own personal story I can help someone out of their own confusion and doubt and into taking care of themselves. And in doing that, by simply taking care of themselves, these people are empowered to see that they really do have more control of their lives and can do much more than they imagined.

I tell a great story in my laughter class about a banker from Texas who was having a heart attack. His 21 year old son was with him and was in a panic. He managed to call 911 and while he and his father were waiting for the ambulance, not knowing what else to do, he started telling his father knock-knock jokes. Well, the father started laughing really hard which in turn released some of the pressure that was building around his heart. When they got to the hospital and told the doctor what they had done, the doctor told the banker and his son that the laughter had saved the banker's life. If he hadn't been laughing and relieving the pressure—he would have been dead by the time they reached they hospital.

One of my favorite financial stories is about an older woman who came to one of my money classes. This woman had always wanted to own real estate, but had given up on the possibility. She decided she could never make enough money and she was too old to start saving. Well, I make a big promise at the beginning of my class that if you do what I say, within a year you can save between ten and twenty thousand dollars. I received a letter from this woman about a year later telling me that not only had she managed to save eighteen thousand dollars, but she had also put a down payment on a co-op. She was so happy with that she was able to accomplish something she never thought she'd be able to do.

Wright

What are the downfalls in life that you are particularly afraid of falling into?

Kaufman

Complacency. One of the things that I am proud of is that none of my speeches are canned or predictable. You could take my laughter therapy class six different times and it would never be the same. Why? Because life changes. Your daughter is going to be a different person at 14 and at 14 and a half. Life happens. But complacency gets in the way of that. You don't notice the nuance and you accept whatever is doled out. It's something we all struggle with. If you're complacent in a relationship you can bet it won't last very long. If you're complacent with your kids, they'll become complacent and be willing to accept mediocrity. The second pit fall is believing that you can make everyone happy all the time. You can't. No one can. It's important to learn to manage our expectations and realize that the best you can ever do is be true to yourself and maintain your integrity

Wright

With all that you have going, being a parent and running your own business, running around the country speaking and all, where does your energy come from?

Kaufman

Sleep! Lack of sleep is probably a leading cause of problems for Americans. I talk about this all of the time. I'm usually asleep by 9:30 and I'm up by quarter of six in the morning feeling rested and energized. Also, I walk my talk and believe that laughter is extremely important. You must see the fun in everything you do. You simply can't get caught up worrying about everything, like the kids and their homework and the ten different places you need to drive them to and the 55 emails you have to answer. These are the realities of your life—of all of our lives, but at the end of the day, instead of being a nervous wreck you can be grateful. One day the kids will be grown and out of the house and the emails will stop and you'll miss all of the activity. Enjoy the moment!

Wright

What about diet and exercise?

Kaufman

Healthy eating habits are extremely important to me. At one point I was obese and had to diet to lose 80 pounds. I had to learn an entirely new set of healthy eating habits—and of course exercise was also very important.

Wright

You lost 80 pounds? That's a whole person.

Kaufman

That is a whole person and I am only five feet tall. I'm a very little person, I mean a very short person.

Wright

What skills have been the most important for you to learn?

Kaufman

Probably the most important corporate skill I've learned and now teach is based upon Daniel Goleman's book, *Emotional Intelligence*. Goleman writes about the importance of being aware of what kind of person you are. I'll use the example of my weight. It seemed obvious to everyone but me that I was obese. I just didn't see myself that way. It was really, really hard to understand that I needed to lose weight. Self-awareness is extremely important. What are you good at? What can you learn to do better? I am constantly enjoying the process of getting better. I enjoy having meetings with my kids to find out how they think I'm doing as a parent. I ask my clients and trainers the same thing. It's great to hear the good stuff, but I also want to hear what I can be doing better. I try not to get defensive about it—and certainly know that I am not perfect at everything (which is a very stressful image to hold of ourselves!). We need learn to wake up every day and see it as a new opportunity to grow and learn. It's easier to say than do sometimes, but it's always worth making the effort. As the Nike commercial says, just do it!

Wright

You said that everyone realized you were obese but you. When you looked in the mirror, what did you see?

Kaufman

I saw a little chunky person. Obesity is the number one epidemic in America and I was not chunky, I was obese but I simply couldn't see it. I've recognized the same thing with some clients who approach me after workshops. They'll tell me that the have a few pounds to lose, but I can see that they are 30, 40, 50 pounds overweight. I see it, but they can't. It's like the guy in the office who drives everyone crazy because he yells all the time. Everyone complains about the yelling and you ask him how he thinks he's doing and he'll say something like, "One thing about me is that I never yell." Denial is an amazing place to live and people do a very good job keeping themselves there.

Sometimes I'll ask parents when the last time was they sat down with their kids to ask them how they thought they were doing as parents. The parents think I'm crazy and wonder why you would ever ask your kids, or spouse or colleagues such a loaded question! Well, you ask because it is really important for you to hear the answer.

Wright

As a parent, how do you teach your children time and stress management?

Kaufman

There's a great saying, "Blessed is the skinned knee." The best thing to do for a kid when they fall down is show them how to get back up.

I teach them about time management using their homework. I'll say, "Your homework needs to be done by 7:00. You make any choice you want, but by 7:00 if it's not done it doesn't get done." I allow them to look at their day and plan it out for themselves giving them tools so that they know what the parameters are, what the repercussions will be if something doesn't get done. And then they make their own choices.

Stress management is easy to teach to kids through laughter therapy because they are so much more receptive to it than adults. Kids also have much better self esteem than most adults. If I tell my 14 year old to go into his room by himself, take off his pajamas or clothes, look in the mirror and tell himself that he's awesome he has no problem doing that. If I go into IBM and tell them to do that they say, "I could never do that." Most people can't give themselves one compliment. The point here is that if you don't feel good about yourself then everything is going to be more difficult for you to cope with and your stress level is going to increase. Have a laugh, think of something good about yourself—it will make things much easier.

Wright

You were talking about the medicinal upsides of laughter and certainly a lot of people that say that. The problem I've found is that they don't know how to teach people how to have fun. How do you teach others to have fun?

Kaufman

You have to take a step back and say, "I'm going to do this because it's going to prolong my life. I'm going to do this because I'm going to have a better quality of life." So I think there is something esoteric about it. People take a pill because it makes them feel better. Well, why not try a good hearty laugh that will also make you feel better? The beauty of laughter therapy is it works even if you fake it! Even if I wake up in the morning in a bad mood, knowing that I have a particularly difficult day ahead if I can stand up, put my hand on my stomach and just start laughing, even if it's fake, I'm going to feel better. You learn by doing and by practicing. You can't learn to do anything well if you don't practice. Some of us need to practice laughing before we really get the hang of it.

I also make a list with my family of things that we do for fun that don't cost money. So when we are looking for something fun to do, we just pull that list out. We're always revising it. You can make a list for yourself—for groups you belong to. A fun list—it's a great tool to have.

Another way to have fun is by helping other people. People will say that they can't add one more thing to their already full plates, but the truth is, this is the thing you'll add that's guaranteed to make you feel better. Try volunteering at a nursing home; it could be one of the most fun experiences if you find the right match. Here are people in their 80's and 90's—think of the amazing stories they have to tell. All you have to do is ask and you'll hear things you never dreamed of that make you feel pretty good and you've cared enough to listen to someone else, which makes them feel good. It's a win-win situation!

There are a million little things you can do to feel good, like eating dessert for dinner every once in a while. Even if you are sticking to a healthy diet, one night of apple pie instead of roast chicken won't hurt you and you'll have fun. Try eating non traditional foods; eat by candlelight; rearrange the furniture, wear different colors, take a new route to work. Sometimes just shaking up the routine and trying something new will make you feel better. It's one of the things we work hard to teach people. Change is good, and fun, and fun is really important!

Wright

I've been married for 26 years now and someone asked my recently what led up to it and how did I meet her and all. I started thinking about that and the truth of the matter is that I was working and I had been eating in this real dull place for days and days and days. One day at lunch I decided to go to the Pizza Hut.

Kaufman

And that's where you met her.

Wright

There she was.

Kaufman

I tell a story about an executive at J.P. Morgan who was very successful and making tons of money. She had everything except she didn't have a significant other in her life. This woman had come to several of my classes and I knew that she really wanted to be a mother, but not a single mother—she wanted to have a child the traditional way and start a family. In this particular class I asked everyone to write their own eulogy—which is a terrific exercise. By writing her eulogy, this woman was able to focus on her goals. She realized that at the age of 40, if she wanted to have a baby, she'd better get moving, but she said she simply didn't have time. So after the class she went home thinking about all of this and she took the bus instead of the subway. Of course she met somebody on the bus and ended up getting married and having a baby. Sometimes life is that simple. We make it so much more complicated than it has to be by looking at all of the negatives instead of all of the possibilities.

I often tell the story of when my ex-husband walked out on me. Everyone in my life was very upset and they would say things like, "Oh my god, Wendy, your life is going to be so hard." Well, that's true, it is hard, and raising kids on your own is very difficult. Interestingly nobody said "This is a great opportunity, now you can do whatever you want to do. You'll be able to start fresh!"

When people lose their jobs not many people will say, "This is so cool. You get to find another job now." Instead they tend towards the negative and their own fears by saying, "It's a terrible economy out there. How are you going to get another job? It's really hard out there. I hope you have a lot of money saved." It's like everyone telling me how hard my life was going to be as a single mother. They took a stressful situation and made it a hundred times worse by being negative instead of turning it around and helping me to see the possibility by saying something like, "How can we help you have fun with this? How can you make this the best situation for you and the children?"

When my dad was getting chemo we didn't sit around with him dwelling on the chemo. Instead we retold very funny stories about when we were kids. The treatment took 6 hours, which would have been unbearable if we had only focused on whether or not the chemo was going to kill or cure him. We focused on the positive and joy that we all shared and it made all of the difference.

Some people are naturally very upbeat and positive and they have the gift of finding the humor in every situation. However, most of us have to learn how to lighten up and have fun with our stress. It makes even the most difficult and trying times much easier to get through.

Wright

I have noticed in the last five years that most of the funerals that I go to are very unlike what they used to be. Now they're celebrations of the person's life and the ministers and people who are delivering eulogies are saying stories that are funny.

Kaufman

Some of the ministers, priests, and rabbis that I do work with will actually screen the people giving the eulogies. They try to keep them from getting too mournful and suggest telling good stories about the person's life. There are also hospitals that are offering memorial services while the people are still living so that they can recall the good times and funny stories along with their families and friends.

I have worked with the widows and widowers of September 11th for the past several years. One of the best things that we did for them was to ask colleagues who worked with people that died that day to write all of the funny stories about their co-workers that they could think of. We made a book of the stories and presented it to the surviving families. We all knew how tragic and awful the loss was and believed that by incorporating humorous stories it would empower the survivors to believe that their lives would be happier one day, and that they would once again experience the fun that had been an important part of their loved ones lives before the events of September 11.

It's an interesting aspect of health and wellness; Exercise, rest, healthy eating are all really important, but without laughter, medical studies show that people are more inclined to fall ill, and their life expectancy is not as long as that of someone who embraces the possibilities of life and takes enjoyment where they can make it.

Many years ago, a man named Victor Frankel made a study of concentration camp survivors. He found that those who gave away their food and told jokes, even though they may have been physically weaker, were more likely to survive than those who didn't. The human spirit is an amazing thing.

We always have a choice. There is good and bad in every situation and there is balance. You can have a nasty commute to work and walk into the office with a bad attitude and a list a mile long of complaints. Or you can be grateful that you made it to the office in one piece, tell a story about something ridiculous a fellow commuter did, and find someone in the office to say hello to, brightening their day. The human spirit is an amazingly resilient thing—if we learn how to fly with it!

About The Author

Wendy Kaufman was born and raised in Westchester, New York. She went to Syracuse University and earned a Bachelor's Degree in Education. Then she completed her Master's Degree in Industrial Psychology from The University of Pennsylvania. Wendy immediately went to work in the Human Resources field for The Hertz Corporation where she concentrated in the compensation department. Making a career transition—she went to Fordham University where she held various positions. Finally, Wendy went to Yeshiva University as the Director of Career Placement. Wendy married and had three children in three and a half years and decided to enter the field of corporate training. During that time, Wendy divorced and faced life's challenges on her own. Now as a single mother her work took a whole new light. She learned to "practice what she preached." After consulting for a number of years for various companies she took the plunge and formed her own company. Balancing Life's Issues, Inc. was started and has grown steadily since its inception. They offer services that include lunch and learns, motivating keynotes, as well as longer training sessions. BLI, Inc. has spoken to IBM, JPMorganChase, Johnson and Johnson, The New York Times, Coach to name a few. Wendy and her group of trainers have a 100% return rate... which means they are always invited back to continue the motivation. Wendy has great plans to continue to have BLI, grow and grow.

Wendy Kaufman

President

Balancing Life Issues, Inc.

14 Saddle Ridge Road

Ossining, New York 10562

Phone: 914-762-9075

Email: wk62@aol.com

Chapter 11

RICHARD W. BUNCH, PH.D., P.T., C.B.E.S.

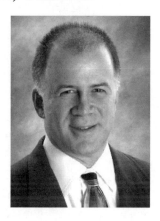

THE INTERVIEW

David E. Wright (Wright)

Today we are talking to Dr. Richard Bunch, a licensed physical therapist with a doctorate degree in anatomy who provides motivational injury prevention and wellness seminars and ergonomic consulting to industries throughout the United States. Dr. Bunch, welcome to *Conversations on Health and Wellness.*

Richard Bunch (Bunch)

Thank you.

Wright

First of all, as a point of clarification, what exactly is ergonomics and how does it relate to wellness?

Bunch

Ergonomics is the study and science of reducing physical and mental stress on a person by altering the work process and environment. Ergonomics has proven to be highly effective for reducing the occurrences of common painful and sometimes disabling conditions related to disorders of the neck, back, shoulders, and carpal tunnel in the wrist. Ergonomic interventions should also increase the efficiency of work and improve productivity. I sincerely believe that ergonomics is an integral part of wellness. We cannot simply engineer out all risk factors of work. Behavior is important, especially lifestyle behaviors that may cause obesity, diabetes, cancer and heart disease. Therefore, my training and consulting services address an integrated approach, combining ergonomics and wellness techniques to obtain optimum health. I call this an *ergo-wellness* approach and it has proven to be very effective for my clients. In essence, this approach creates a win-win situation for both the employer and the employee. The employer benefits from a healthier and more productive work force and the employee benefits from a better quality life.

Wright

Why do you travel and use this integrated approach with industries rather than, like most clinicians today, work in a clinic on a full time basis?

Bunch

Well, it boils down to whether you want to address the cause of most health problems that afflict people today or simply treat the symptoms. My philosophy changed from the traditional reactive approach in physical therapy to a much more proactive, holistic approach as a result of my early experiences treating injured employees. For instance, many years ago I evaluated a young man with chronic, disabling back pain, who in less that three years, had already undergone five back surgeries! During this time period he had become an alcoholic and addicted to Percodan, a narcotic. Because of a personality change related to pain and his inability to have a normal relationship, his wife ended up divorcing him. All of these terrible things started with simple back pain and evolved into these serious consequences in a relatively short time span. I remember asking him, "Sir, in the first year you had back pain and before you had your first surgery, didn't anybody ask what type of work you were involved in and how you performed your job? Did anyone show you how to perform the duties of your job without re-injuring your back? For example, did anyone show you how to work in non-stressful postures and how to perform posture relief exercises? His response was "No" to every one of those questions. This man was a pipe-fitter, a job that involved heavy manual labor. The cause of his back problems, poor lifting techniques and prolonged, awkward work postures were never addressed by the treating clinicians. It then dawned on me from this case and unfortunately, too many others that followed, that traditional reactive medical treatment was simply ineffective in most cases. In fact, I became to feel that not addressing the cause of a condition related to work and lifestyles was tantamount to malpractice. Think about it. Administering passive modalities such as hot packs and electrical stimulation, injecting the body with cortisone, prescribing drugs such as anti-inflammatory pain medications and muscle relaxers are all methods that address symptoms and not the cause. So I decided to go out to the workplace and look at jobs and how people were actually performing the jobs. I assessed the effects of work postures, force, and repetition on the human body. I also became focused on helping people lose weight, learn effective stress coping techniques and become more physically fit. I became, without knowing it, involved in ergonomics when most people weren't even talking about ergonomics. Since then I've had so many great results from integrating ergonomic principles with wellness concepts. By using this integrative approach, I now feel that I am addressing the real cause of the majority of problems that most people face in this country.

Wright

So what is your basic philosophy or primary principle about health that you want to convey to the people?

Bunch

Well, I want people to truly understand that most bad things that will happen to their health today and in the future will stem from their own lifestyle and work behaviors. With today's modern medicine major diseases such as bubonic plague or malaria are no longer afflicting us. We are dying prematurely from cancer, complications of diabetes, heart disease, and strokes. We are suffering from arthritis and other musculoskeletal problems. Even if we live long, many of the retirement years, a time when we should really be enjoying life, are too often, years of suffering and disability. Ironically, 90% or more of these conditions are totally prevented by changing lifestyle habits and knowing how to take better care of ourselves. For example, in the year 2002, 20 million people in the United States suffered from diabetes. Ninety percent of these diabetic patients are Type II diabetics, the acquired form, which means that this disease was caused primarily by poor lifestyle behaviors related to overeating, becoming obese, and lack of exercise. We can have a tremendous positive impact on this costly disease by simply exercising and adhering to proper nutrition. Yet, most people wait until they have this disease, which at this time has no cure, and then become dependent on drugs such as insulin. More often, diabetics only begin to exercise and watch the foods they eat after being frightened into these behavioral changes by an onset of a very serious, life threatening disease. This is a typical human behavior. We wait until an event that threatens our quality life to occur before we take actions that would have ironically prevented the problem in the first place.

Cancer is another example of a disease that many people erroneously do not view as lifestyle related. One of the leading oncologists in the country correlated risk factors associated with this dreaded disease to three primary factors: poor nutrition, psychological stress, and lack of exercise. All three of these risk factors are typically consequences of behavior, not a germ or virus! Likewise, most arthritic conditions that disable people involve *degenerative* arthritis. Degenerative arthritis, in actuality, is nothing more than wearing out joints in the body, typically related to being overweight (overloading the joints) and poor muscle protection of the joints from being out of shape.

So the answer is becoming increasingly clear that proper nutrition, weight control, and regular exercise is essential to good health. This means that people have to really get serious about taking control of their lives and commit to making health their number one priority in life.

Wright

What are some everyday common lifestyle habits that people should be aware of that increase their risk for health problems?

Bunch

Well, some of them are quite surprising. For example, if you skip breakfast every day, you are twice as likely to become obese, acquire Type II diabetes and have cardiovascular disease. If you are under chronic stress, you are more likely to become ill as stress compromises the immune system by accelerating the depletion of vitamins and minerals in the body. Another common lifestyle problem today is inadequate sleep. Most Americans do not get eight hours of sleep. They get much less, on average, six hours of sleep. Lack of sleep is also related to compromising the immune system. On top of all this people are not eating properly and they are certainly not exercising enough. We're eating foods that are highly processed carbohydrates. Much of what we eat today is not organic and healthy. The result: A compromised immune system and obesity with all its related terrible medical problems that shorten life or destroy the quality of life.

I mentioned that lack of exercise is a big issue today. The American Heart Association announced many years ago that moderate exercise for as little as 30 minutes a day, just four days a week will cut a person's risk of heart disease by as much as 50 percent. Yet, many people will not even do that! Studies also show that moderate exercise 30 minutes a day and losing only 7% of your body weight will cut the risk of Type II Diabetes by more than 60%!

So these are all the things that I feel people don't fully understand. When I conduct my motivational seminars, I try to motivate people to take action, to make a disciplined commitment to improving health everyday by making them understand the consequences of their poor lifestyle behaviors.

Wright

How is your message or approach different from most others in the health field?

Bunch

Well, I hope I am one among a growing population of healthcare providers that are becoming focused on the total proactive or holistic approach. Too many clinicians today limit their practice to evaluating a person's condition and treating the symptoms. I feel this is a totally inadequate treatment for the types of health problems we face today in modern America. I tenaciously avoid that reactive approach. In addition to assessing a person's health problem, I complete an analysis of what their jobs require and their lifestyle habits. I want to know all the factors that could be contributing to or causing a medical problem. I want to make sure that the person knows what corrective actions to take, how to improve his or her physical fitness level, and how to prevent medical problems from occurring again. This is a far cry from telling a person that they need to come see me on an ongoing basis for passive treatment modalities. In my opinion, we should never make people feel that they must depend on healthcare providers for maintaining optimum health. They must learn to do that for themselves. People need to fully understand the role of proper nutrition and exercise in maintaining optimum health. They need to know how to combat stress in a healthy manner rather than by using drugs or by chronic overeating.

As an ergonomic consultant, I have also learned a lot from safety professionals, especially those who practice behavioral-based safety. I am one of the biggest fans of safety professionals because they can effectively address the root causes of many of the injuries and illnesses that affect the working population today. This is why I joined the American Society of Safety Engineers (ASSE), and provide seminars at national ASSE conferences. By providing ergo-wellness facilitator training to safety specialists, I can help these professionals become more effective in injury prevention and improving employee fitness. In many cases, and I mean this sincerely, a good safety professional can do more for a person than many healthcare providers can. This relates, again, to providing the real cure through *prevention* and not just treating symptoms.

As a practicing physical therapist, I can bring clinical knowledge to the field and share that knowledge with people while I am conducting ergonomic assessments. I think of the work site as an extension of my clinic and my ergo-wellness approach as a medical treatment directed at the root cause of the majority of problems affecting people today.

Wright

Have you had any life experiences that made you want to travel and focus so much on helping people improve the quality of their lives through ergonomic consulting and seminars?

Bunch

Well, it seems like a lot of professional speakers commonly relate to some type of life changing event that helped mold their particular method or approach in training. I guess I am no exception. In 1990, I had a horrible event where I was in the wrong place at the wrong time. I was carjacked at gunpoint by two men and forced into the trunk of my car where I was held for more than 9 hours. You can imagine I was pretty much traumatized and worried about what was going to happen to me. I ended up in Galveston, Texas where I was taken out of the trunk of the car and beat up and left for dead. A night fisherman fortunately rescued me. I tell this story to my audiences only because I want people to know what goes through a person's mind when the reality of death is at hand. When I was in the trunk of my car, the last thing I thought about was how much money

I made, the type of clothes I wore, or what kind of car I drove. You know, all the stupid material, status-related things that people too often get hung up on these days. Instead, the only thing my mind focused on was praying to God to allow me one more opportunity to see and hold my wife and children again. I remembered thinking how wonderful it would be just to be able to spend a single day with them again or even just to see them for a second. This experience made it painfully clear how important those relationships were in my life. Unfortunately, I have also seen this same life-changing reaction in terminally ill patients. You can see that their whole attitude had changed from focusing on material things and trivial matters to what was, is, and always will be the most valuable thing in their lives, their health. But, having a life threatening disease or event is a horrible way for a person to learn that they should have spent more time with the family, worried less, exercised more, and eaten healthier. So I take that message to the people around the country and world with the hope that I can motivate them to make healthy changes in their lives that can improve the quality of life's experiences and enrich the relationships with family and friends.

I sincerely believe that the basis for most illnesses and poor quality of life stems from unhealthy behaviors that stem from flawed priorities in life. A person will typically think, "I'll do what I need to do for my job, my spouse, and children first, and if there is any time left over I'll take care of myself. That attitude may seem laudable at first glance, but it is basically flawed, and in most cases, harmful. What I teach people to do is flip that "priority pyramid," placing oneself back at the top, and in effect begin to think, "I'm going to take care of myself first so that I'll be a better employee, a better spouse, and a better parent." By actually moving health up to the number one priority in life, a person will be around longer to take care of these entities. I tell people, it is not hard to become disabled or even die. The hard part relates to the immeasurable suffering and hardships that your disability or death will cause the very people you want to protect and love.

Wright

As both a clinician and a professional speaker, how do you feel that your background has helped you to effectively motivate people to make work and lifestyle changes that have a positive effect on health?

Bunch

Well, from the very issue of being a clinician, I have the benefits of clinical experience of seeing the injuries and illnesses after they happen in a traditional clinical environment. And then as a speaker and consultant, I can relate my clinical experience to people in a manner that will clearly clarify why they need to take steps now to improve health. Too many great doctors and therapists and their clinics are doing excellent clinical jobs, but they don't have time in their clinics to educate people.

Wright

What do you think are the biggest health problem trends today?

Bunch

Well, the biggest health problem trends today can be addressed on two levels. We have a big problem with an aging, deconditioned, obese baby boomer generation. And then we have a different kind of problem with the younger, deconditioned, computer-game based sedentary generation. These kids today are growing up being babysat by computer games. They are becoming couch potatoes at a very early age. Even our country sponsors such behavior by not requiring schools to provide physical education anymore. Parents are too often poor role models and do not encourage their children to eat right and exercise daily. Consequently, about twenty-seven percent of children are overweight. We are experiencing about 1,000 percent increase in diabetes since 1900 because of processed foods. The cost of diabetes in 2002 alone was approximately $132 billion. Therefore, the biggest medical problems we're seeing right now relate to an epidemic of poor physical fitness and obesity.

Another important issue is that many people do not understand the connection of stress to health. Overeating is a common side product of stress. People have found that eating produces sedating hormones. People, therefore, use food as a drug to cope with stress. Studies show that stress reduces a human's capacity to retain vitamins and minerals. Combine this knowledge with the fact that Americans are ingesting poor quality foods that are high in sugar and fat and low in vitamins and minerals. This leads to all kinds of illnesses and diseases and even cancer. Now, if you add other unhealthy habits such as smoking, drinking too much alcohol, drugs, breathing polluted air, and drinking bad water, your probability of getting cancer significantly increases.

Wright

Do you really think that the majority of disabling conditions, including the common joint aches and pains that people complain about today, result from their lifestyles and not just from genetics or just the aging process?

Bunch

Yes, I really do. The scientific studies support that as well. I am not ignoring the issue of genetics. But the fact is that we cannot change who our parents are. We can only change lifestyles. Consider for example, spinal problems, a common disabling condition today. A virus or germ does not selectively cause your lower cervical (neck) disk or lower lumbar (back) disc to degenerate or rupture. Such occurrences are overwhelmingly related to mechanical stress from prolonged awkward postures, poor material handling techniques (e.g., bad lifting technique), and declining physical fitness.

Many jobs today involve working at a computer. If you analyze office workers, most of them sit slumped in a chair with their heads projected forward of their bodies. Medical studies show that when the head is positioned forward of the body, spinal disc pressure significantly increases at the base of the neck. Therefore, it is no surprise that the most common site of disc surgery in the neck is at the lowest level, around the sixth and seventh neck vertebrae. An even more frightful medical problem can occur among computer users who wear progressive lens, bifocals and trifocals. These workers typically tilt their chins up to look through the bottom lens of their glasses. When tilting their chins up, especially while projecting their heads forward in a slumped posture, there is significant compression on vertebral joints, called facet joints. This can lead to significant neck pain and headaches. This same posture will compress the vertebral arteries that travel up the vertebral column of the neck to enter the brain via an opening at the base of the skull. The vertebral arteries make a 90-degree turn over the first vertebra of the neck in order to pass under the skull into an opening for the brainstem. Damage to these arteries occur at this vulnerable location, where the arteries become sandwiched between the skull and vertebrate while a person is titling the chin up to look through the lower lens of their glasses. Mechanical compression and compromised blood flow at this location can lead to spasms of these arteries and severe headaches - a common complaint of office workers. Long term consequences of chronic irritation of the vertebral arteries are speculative. However, it is reasonable to suspect that chronic mechanical compression of these arteries may lead to a buildup of plaque that can increase the risk of a stroke.

Now, consider heart disease. Changing behavior can definitely help reduce this potentially devastating problem. Too much cholesterol and triglycerides in the blood are well known and risk factors associated are with poor nutritional habits and lack of exercise. We also know that cardiovascular diseases that result from irritation to the linings of the blood vessels can be related to insufficient vitamin B complex in our diet. Vitamin B deficiencies lead to an elevation of an amino acid called homocysteine in the blood stream that is responsible for this problem. Unfortunately, vitamin B deficiencies are not uncommon in the United States since almost all vitamin B complex is found in green leafy vegetables, a diet that people are just not simply eating enough of these days. The other issue in relation to heart disease is that more and more people are suffering from high levels of cholesterol. Some people simply produce too much cholesterol by the liver and need to take medication to get their cholesterol under control despite exercise and proper diets. However, there are risk factors for high cholesterol related to poor diets and insufficient exercise. For many years, diet-related high cholesterol was thought to be the result of eating foods high in fat, a view that led to the low fat diet craze. Now, most people know, if they read the latest diet books such as the *South Beach Diet, Atkins Diet, Sugar Busters,* and the G.I. *Diet,* that processed carbohydrates plays a large role in this problem. Excess carbohydrates that have a high glycemic index (i.e., that are broken down into sugar quickly), are converted to triglycerides by insulin and increase the levels of serum LDL, the bad carrier of cholesterol that helps plug up arteries. So again, we need to go back to root cause of all these problems and address <u>behaviors</u> such as poor nutrition and lack of exercise. Reducing processed carbohydrates and avoiding harmful fats in our diets has a powerful impact on the blood serum levels and weight loss. In addition, exercising regularly is essential for helping the body metabolize glucose and fats that can form plaques in the blood vessels that later lead to strokes and heart attacks.

Wright

Although I know you have respect for competent professionals in all types of health care professions, you have indicated that health care today is too reactive and not proactive enough. Could you clarify your position and indicate how our health care system needs to change to better address the problems in the years to come?

Bunch

Yes, the biggest problem with medicine in the country today is that medicine has become a business. We have too many clinicians that are in the business of medicine and not in the practice of medicine. It's not uncommon to hear patients complain how they waited in a clinic for one, two, or more hours to be finally seen by a healthcare provider for only seven to ten minutes. I do not know how we can evaluate patients effectively, address the root causes of the health problem, and provide an effective treatment plan that addresses the cause of the problem in such a short time period. If both lifestyle and work behaviors contribute to many of the health problems today, as we know they do, how can any clinician analyze and effectively treat these issues in such a short time period? On top of this, insurance companies do not want to spend money on proactive wellness programs that will prevent these problems from happening in the first place. Instead, we find insurance companies paying for expensive medical treatments of problems that could have been easily prevented by a proactive wellness program. I feel that healthcare providers and insurance risk managers should be trained in ergonomics and wellness, as these fields have become so important in alleviating modern day health problems. If we could alter the way we deliver medical care in this fashion, the results would be quite spectacular.

Wright

You know vitamin and mineral supplements appear to be gaining increasing favor by medical practitioners and lay people alike. I know you're in favor of vitamin supplements. Why do you think we need to take vitamin supplements today, and do we need them if we eat healthy?

Bunch

Nutritional supplements are nothing more than a form of insurance to help protect people from poor diets and stressful lifestyles. If we still lived on farms, ate organically grown food, and lived a slower, stress-free life, then taking supplements would probably not be needed. Poor nutrition and chronic stress rob us of natural vitamins and minerals. It is ironic that we are seeing vitamin deficiency related illnesses increase today in our modern society. Studies have recently shown an increase in cases of rickets from vitamin D deficiencies, especially in areas of the country where there is little exposure to the sun. We have documented heart disease related to vitamin B deficiencies and an increased risk of cancer from low diet levels of a trace mineral called selenium. In today's fast food, high stress world, it is obvious that there should be a lot more focus on how nutrition affects our health.

Wright

You recommend a certain vitamin regimen and minerals based on well-documented research in several well-known publications. In a nutshell, what are they, why are they important, and what are the precautions for taking vitamins and minerals?

Bunch

Well, there are a lot of vitamins out there, and I cannot obviously address all of them. But let me mention a few that I think are very important and have been receiving tremendous attention by health-care providers. Research suggests that many over-the-counter multiple vitamin supplements simply do not provide sufficient dosages for optimum effects in today's environment. That's why you can buy some of these multiple vitamins over the counter so cheaply. The following list of vitamins, minerals and coenzymes appear to have good scientific support for effectiveness in reducing a person's risk of serious diseases:

Vitamin A - 5,000 mg
Vitamin C - 400 – 800 mg
Vitamin E -1,000 to 1,200 IU
Selenium – 200 mcg
Vitamin B complex (100, 150 or 150 complex)
Alpha Lipoic Acid – 300 mg
Coenzyme Q10 – 100 – 120 mg

One will note that these dosage levels are considerably more than what is found in a multiple vitamin that offers only the recommended daily allowance (RDA). The higher dosages given are considered "optimum" for preventing diseases including cancer and heart disease. Vitamins A, E, and C are antioxidants that help to fight off free radicals associated with aging, cancer and heart disease. Vitamin C, made famous by Dr. Linus Pauling, is extremely important for bolstering the immune system and fighting viruses. By the way, the first vitamin that is depleted from the body by stress is Vitamin C. B complex, consisting mainly of B_6, B_{12}, and Folic acid, is extremely important for helping to prevent heart disease. Folic acid also offers the additional benefit of helping pregnant women reduce their risk of neural tube birth defects called spina bifida. Cardiologists often prescribe folic acid to patients after they have heart attacks. In my opinion, why wait to have a heart attack to prescribe something we know that helps prevent heart attacks.

Co-enzyme Q10 is a powerful antioxidant that also helps prevent heart disease. Alpha lipoic acid, often referred to as the universal antioxidant, plays a role in helping stabilize blood glucose levels. This provides obvious benefits related to adult onset diabetes. Certainly, there are many other nutritional supplements worthy of mention, such as the flaxseed and fish oils for heart health, calcium for bone strength, specific herbs, etc, but this interview would never end if we tried to address them all. There are volumes of books written about nutritional supplements that people can acquire from any local bookstore. I personally recommend *Dr. Atkin's Vita-Nutrient Solution* by Robert Atkins, M.D., *The Vitamin Revolution in Health Care* by Michael Janson, M.D., and *The Real Vitamin and Mineral Book* by Lieberman and Bruning. People should read about nutritional supplements and gain a better understanding of how important these supplements are to health.

In regard to precautions, people should always avoid taking extremely large amounts of vitamins as they can have harmful side effects at such levels. People have different body chemistries and may have existing medical problems that will be adversely affected by certain supplements. Therefore, people with medical problems should always consult with their medical doctors first before taking supplements, especially when the amounts exceed the recommended daily allowance (RDA). There are physiological effects of nutrients that should be understood and respected. For instance, vitamin E should not be taken prior to any major surgery because vitamin E reduces blood-clotting time. Young children should not take adult dosages of vitamins and minerals. Adult level iron, for example, is toxic to a young child. That's why there are pediatric vitamins available on the market. There are many herbs being pedaled on the market today. Some have medical research that supports their usefulness. However, many people do not understand that herbs are drugs and can be harmful. Marijuana, for example is a herb. Many herbs have not been validated as being effective and one should approach herbs with caution until more research supports any alleged benefits. So there are precautions one must consider when taking supplements and understanding how to take nutritional supplements is important to everybody. To be on the safe side, I always recommend that people should check with their medical doctor prior to taking nutritional supplements.

Wright

Well, what a wonderful conversation! You probably feel like we haven't even covered half of what you know about the subject, but this has just really been a great discussion on health. Today we have been talking to Richard W. Bunch, PhD, and physical therapist. He is an ergonomic specialist, a professional injury prevention and wellness speaker/trainer, and he is a licensed physical therapist with a Doctorate Degree in human anatomy, and as we have found out this afternoon, he is full of information on health and wellness. Richard, thank you so much for being with us today on *Conversations on Health and Wellness*.

Bunch

Thank you, David, I appreciated this opportunity to speak to you and share this information with readers.

About The Author

Dr. Bunch is a highly sought after nationally renown public speaker, author, and consultant on the topics of wellness and ergonomics. As a clinician, ergonomic consultant and motivational injury prevention and wellness speaker he has helped over 900,000 employees reduce their risks to musculoskeletal injuries such as neck, back, shoulder and carpal tunnel problems, improve fitness, control stress, lose weight and significantly reduce their risk of diabetes, cancer and heart disease. His training programs have directly helped industries reduce medical problems by as much as 78%. Dr. Bunch attended the U.S. Military Academy at West Point, and later became a licensed physical therapist and ergonomic specialist with a medical Ph.D. in Human Anatomy. He is a member of the National Speakers Association (NSA). As a native Louisianan, based out of new Orleans, Dr. Bunch is well noted for blending Cajun humor in his seminars with the belief that along with all the wonderful health tips he addresses, that laughter is still good medicine.

Richard W. Bunch, Ph.D., P.T., C.B.E.S.

Phone: 800-414-2174

E-mail: Bunchisr@AOL.com

Chapter 12

Maria Perno Goldie, RDH, BA, MS

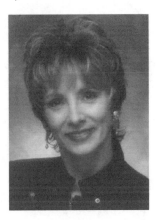

THE INTERVIEW

David E. Wright (Wright)

Today we are talking to Maria Perno Goldie. A noted researcher, author, and speaker, Maria presents seminars nationally and internationally on topics such as women's health and wellness, the oral/systemic link, and periodontal disease. She has appeared on network radio and television interviews regarding the link between periodontal disease and systemic disease and in the *Fox Health Network* WEBMD TV, *The Cutting Edge Medical Report*. Maria is a quoted expert in *Women's Doctors Guide to Heath and Healing*. Maria is a member of the National Advisory Committee for the Robert Wood Johnson Foundation's Smoking Cessation Leadership Central Program, my goodness that's a long word, The International Federation of Dental Hygienists', The National Speakers' Association, and the National Women's Health Resource Center, Women's Health Advisory Counsel. As a board member of the Dental Health Foundation, she helps underserved communities and contributes to the education and policy making of a number of organizations. Maria served as 1997 - 1998 president of the American Dental Hygienists' Association, (ADHA). Welcome to our program today, Maria!

Maria Perno Goldie (Goldie)
Well, thank you very much.

Wright
As the owner of Seminars for Women's Health, you travel national and internationally to present seminars. Tell me about your seminars, where you go, what you present.

Goldie
Most of my presentations are in the United States, although I do travel internationally as well. I have presented in Canada, Italy, Australia, New Zealand, Germany, Sweden, and am on my way to Spain. My audience is mostly health care providers and primarily oral health care providers such as dental hygienists and dentists. What I do is marry oral health and general health. One of the ways that I do this is by talking specifically about women's health and sex-based medicine, which gained my interest a number of years ago when I was working on my Masters Degree.

Wright
So, what peaked your interest in women's health?

Goldie
I'm a dental hygienist as I said, and 99.9% of the individuals in our profession are women, and most times dental hygienists make up my audience. Even if there are male dental hygienists or dentists in attendance, they clinically treat women clients about 50% of the time! So, I thought while I'm doing my presentations on oral health, if I talked about issues that were of specific importance to women, they would probably be of interest to men as well. While I was working toward my Master's Degree, I wrote my thesis on women's health issues and really started to see, from a biological perspective, the difference between men and women as far as health care delivery. So, even though I teach mostly women's health, I strive to make people understand the differences between men and women in this completely new area of study called Sex Based Biology or Sex Based Medicine.

Wright

Well, I go to a dental hygienist when she can corral me, but I never knew what a dental hygienist was, and what role she plays, or in this case, maybe *he* would play in total health.

Goldie

As I mentioned, the profession is primarily women, but we definitely try to recruit men into the profession. Dental hygienists are licensed oral health professionals who focus on preventing and treating oral diseases-both to protect teeth and gums, and to protect clients'/patients' total health. They are graduates of accredited dental hygiene education programs in colleges and universities, and must take written and clinical exams before they are allowed to practice. In addition to treating clients/patients directly, dental hygienists also work as educators, researchers, and administrators. A dental hygienist can work in many other settings, such as: in a public health setting; with a corporate entity; or as a change agent in a variety of roles. The primary role of a dental hygienist is to teach a client/patient how to take care of their oral health to make sure they are "totally" or systemically healthy. Each state has its own specific regulations and the range of services performed by dental hygienists varies from one state to another. As part of dental hygiene services, dental hygienists may perform the following:

- perform oral health care assessments that include reviewing clients' health history, dental charting, oral cancer screening, and taking and recording blood pressure;
- expose, process, and interpret dental X-rays;
- remove plaque and calculus (tartar)-soft and hard deposits-from above and below the gumline;
- apply cavity-preventive agents such as fluorides and sealants to the teeth;
- teach clients proper oral hygiene techniques to maintain healthy teeth and gums;
- counsel clients about plaque control and developing individualized at-home oral hygiene programs; and
- counsel clients on the importance of good nutrition for maintaining optimal oral health.

There is a large quantity of information from the Surgeon General's Report on Oral Health, as well as many other studies that show that if you have oral disease, it can affect the rest of your body. A case in point, if you have periodontal disease and are pregnant, there is a higher risk of having a preterm, low birth weight baby. You may be at increased risk for cardiovascular and heart disease. If you have periodontal infection and you are a diabetic.... that can be a double-edged sword. Uncontrolled blood sugar can exacerbate periodontitis, and periodontal infection can make it more difficult to control sugar and insulin levels. So there are many links, and a dental hygienist works with a client/patient to teach them how to be responsible for their own health care, and to become partners in prevention. We're moving more from the reparative model, in other words fixing problems, to the Wellness Model, where we promote health and wellness. The focus is on prevention, rather than treatment, of disease. I might see someone in my clinical practice every three months, four months, or six months, but they need to perform a great deal of self care in the interim. They can't rely solely on me to keep their oral health at its optimal level, rather, we are partners in their care. So basically, dental hygienists are preventive oral health care specialists.

Wright

So what is the American Dental Hygienists' Association (ADHA) of which you were a President in '97, '98?

Goldie

The American Dental Hygienists' Association is an organization that is a member-based, and ADHA represents the interest of dental hygienists. It was formed in 1923, so it's been around for a long time, and it's the largest organization representing over 120,000 registered/licensed dental hygienists in the United States. Our mission at ADHA is to improve the public's total health, ensuring that they have access to quality oral health care, increasing awareness of the cost-effective benefits of prevention, promoting the highest standards of dental hygiene education, licensure, practice and research and representing and promoting the interests of dental hygienists. We achieve this by increasing the public's awareness of the benefits of prevention, such as cost effective benefits and systemic health benefits. And ADHA wants to ensure that the highest standards of dental hygiene education are met so that we can be educating and graduating individuals that are qualified to work on the public. We want to make sure that when someone goes to a dental hygienist, they are encountering someone that is a licensed, qualified professional. ADHA is a national, tripartite organization, with constituent (state) and component (local) levels of the organization. ADHA strives to not only help the members, but ultimately help the public as well.

Wright

You mentioned the link between oral and the total health. So what is the link between the two?

Goldie

Well, again going back to the Surgeon General's report, the Surgeon General has reported that a person cannot be healthy unless they have optimal oral health. We now have evidence to support the claim that if somebody has periodontal infection, the infection can affect the rest of his or her body. First of all, bacteria are the cause of periodontal infection, and the oral bacteria can travel from the mouth through the blood stream and affect different parts of the body. That's the first suggested mechanism of systemic involvement. Another theory is that whether you have an infection in your finger, in your ear, or in your mouth, the body's immune response kicks in, and that immune response sets off a cascade of events starting with inflammation, going on to cause many different things to happen in the body. One thing, as I mentioned earlier, is that this process can possibly increase the incidence of preterm, low birth weight babies by starting premature labor. Another thing to keep in mind is heart disease, the number one killer of men and women. Heart disease is now thought to have an infection or inflammatory based component. It has been suggested by researchers that periodontal disease "kick starts" the immune system and might contribute to increased plaque buildup in the blood vessels, in the arteries, and in the veins. Not the same kind of plaque, or biofilm that is in the mouth, but the type that forms from fatty materials in our cardiovascular system. Another connection between oral and systemic diseases is respiratory disease. There have been studies conducted in nursing homes where individuals are not receiving any oral health care, or inadequate care, and these individuals are inhaling harmful oral bacteria on a regular basis. There have been studies where the researchers have isolated oral bacteria in the lungs of these nursing home residents with pneumonia and bronchitis. As I mentioned earlier, there is also the diabetes link. These are just a couple of the links between oral disease and general disease throughout the body.

Wright

What is sex-based medicine? I've never heard of that term before.

Goldie

Well, many people haven't heard the term, and many will say "gender-based medicine" instead of "sex based medicine." Gender used to be the politically correct thing to say in all instances. When we talk about something that's sex based, we mean looking at the sex of an individual, whether they are biologically male or female. When we look at men & women in society, we are looking at "gender" roles. Sex based medicine is a completely new field of study and whether you are a man or a woman, your biological makeup is different (surprise!) and therefore, your predilection for certain diseases might be different as well.

We know, for instance, that men and women differ when giving directions! If you ask a man or woman directions to a certain place, you might get to that place, but you're going to get there in a very different way or with different directions depending on the sex of the person giving the directions. Women appear to rely on landmarks to navigate their environments, whereas men tend to use compass directions. If you hand a man or a woman a remote control, you're going to see very different actions there, as well! We do not need research to observe this, but why these differences occur is based on science. The brain of a man and women is different, and the way each sex uses their brain is different. Imaging studies of the living brain indicate that in women, neurons on both sides of the brain are activated when they are listening, while in men, neurons on only one side of the brain are activated. I wonder if that is why men can tune us out so well!

Our hearts are also different, ... they function differently. Women and men have different signs and symptoms of heart and cardiovascular diseases (CVD) in some cases and women typically develop CVD up to 10 years later than men. Diseases like depression, eating disorders, autoimmune diseases, and osteoporosis affect far more women more than men. With autoimmune diseases, three of four individuals affected are women. Certain kinds of pain medication work better on a man than a woman and vice versa. The class of drugs called kappa opiates is far more effective in relieving pain in women than in men.

So there are many physiological things that happen and will happen differently in our bodies depending on whether we are a man or a woman, and there's an entire area of research devoted to this topic. The Society for Women's Health Research (http://www.womenshealth.org/) has been a pioneer in this arena. The theory is that, in the future, part of the risk assessment process will involve asking the question... is this person a man or a woman? And that will make a difference on how they are treated, the type of drugs they are given, the quantity of drug, etc. Some predict that some day there may be different toothpastes developed for men & women!

Wright

So what do you wish to accomplish by spreading the word about oral health and women's health?

Goldie

There are many dental hygienists around the world. There are a number of individuals who will see their dentist or dental hygienist on a regular basis, but maybe not any other health care professional. They have gotten into the habit of having preventive oral health care checkups, but maybe have not done the same with medical checks . A number of dental hygienists will take a blood pressure before an appointment. If a dental hygienist should see signs of diabetes, eating disorders, tobacco use, or high blood pressure, they are in a position to make appropriate referrals. Consequently my goal is to educate dental hygienists and other health care professionals about not just oral health but also women's health, sex based medicine, and how to incorporate all of these issues to insure total wellness.

Wright

Will there be a correlation between bad dental hygiene and something like blood pressure?

Goldie

Definitely there could be, and there are ongoing studies looking into not only high blood pressure, but all known risk factors for heart disease, such as: stress, hostility, diabetes, smoking, weight, blood lipids, inflammatory markers such as C reactive protein, family history, diet, alcohol and physical activity. We know that most people that have periodontal infection have poor oral hygiene, but that may not necessarily predispose them to a systemic disease. We must take into consideration other risk factors. However, if one has periodontal disease or a periodontal infection, we do know that it could increase their risk of heart disease. We do not have any specific proof that oral disease or bacteria *causes* heart disease, but we do know it can increase risk. Many people do not realize that what happens in your mouth can definitely affect the rest of your body. For instance, if a dental hygienist has a pregnant woman in their chair, they would treat that woman differently than someone that's not pregnant. The kinds of things that we would talk to them about would be different, such as how *their* oral health may be affecting their fetus or could possibly cause preterm delivery. The other thing to educate them about is the infectious nature of not only periodontal bacteria, but also the bacteria that cause tooth decay. A mom can actually transmit strep mutans bacteria to her child when the child is born. That child would then be at a higher risk for tooth decay than someone whose mother has a healthy mouth. So, trying to educate a pregnant woman about keeping her mouth clean and keeping these bacteria at bay will definitely help the child later in life, and it's very easily accomplished. As an example, studies have been performed on pregnant women from six months of pregnancy to when the child is six months old. The pregnant women used either chlorhexidine rinse (an antimicrobial rinse), or chewing gum that contained Xylitol, which is a sugar substitute. The study showed that the pregnant women actually decreased the numbers of bacteria present in their mouths, and therefore decreased the numbers that are transmitted to their child. Since oral bacteria can be transmitted, one must be cautious of kissing, sharing food, or food utensils, sharing items like toothbrushes, and so on. Because you're not going to stop a mom from tasting a child's food, or kissing her child, we need to do the next best thing...explain to them that when they are healthy, they are not transmitting harmful bacteria to their child.... I think they will definitely listen!

Wright

The long name that I stumbled over in your bio ...I'm going to try it again because I want to ask you a question about it. What is the *National Advisory Committee for the Robert Wood Johnson Foundation's Smoking Cessation Leadership Center Program*, and by the way, what is your role in it?

Goldie

I am a board member of this organization, and I too have difficulty saying that name quickly! This is a committee that is housed in the University of California, San Francisco. It is a national advisory committee of the Robert Wood Johnson Foundation, and the Smoking Cessation Leadership part might be a little bit misleading. It's really about Tobacco Cessation Leadership, in other words, helping folks stop using all forms of tobacco products. What this organization is doing is partnering with health care organizations throughout the country to help people stop using tobacco. And how can we do this? This committee's goal is action-oriented, not to study things or conduct research projects, but to implement programs that help people *stop* smoking and using tobacco products. An example would be the partnership created between the Smoking Cessation Leadership Center and the American Dental Hygienists Association. This partnership has resulted in resources to help dental hygiene professionals on the state and the local level to reach every dental hygienist in the country. It is a kind of "train the trainer program," where leaders are being trained to coach other dental hygienists to spend three minutes with their clients asking them very simple questions. An example of this scenario would be:

DH: "Do you use tobacco?"
Client "Yes, I do."
DH: "What type of tobacco do you use?"
Client "Well, "I smoke cigarettes" or "I use spit tobacco" or whatever the case may be. DH: "Would you like to stop?"
Client "Well, I'd love to but I've tried and it's very difficult and I can't seem to achieve success."

Then the dental hygienist can implement a tobacco cessation program if they have one set up in the office, or they can simply refer that individual to a tobacco cessation quit line. Quit lines are available in almost every state. We are now in the process of getting a national quit line, and this is the place where someone can call and have invaluable resources that will help them to stop using tobacco. The main reason that health care professionals, such as physicians, nurses, dentists, and dental hygienists do not institute tobacco cessation programs is (they say) they don't have the time. And as smoking is the largest preventable cause of death in the country, and in the world, a life can possibly be saved in one minute to three minutes. When stated in these terms, I don't think anybody can then say, "I don't have the time." The ultimate goal of this program is to have *every* dental hygienist in *every* office take a minute to three minutes, ask these questions, and make the appropriate referrals. The realistic goal set is 50% of all dental hygienists.

Go to: <http://smokingcessationleadership.ucsf.edu/> or www.adha.org> for more information.

Wright

So what can consumers of health care do to attain and maintain health?

Goldie

I think one of the things they need to do is to educate themselves and stay informed. They should also collaborate with their health care providers, whether it's their dental hygienist, dentist, physician, or nurse practitioner. Whoever it may be. By partnering with health care providers and learning how to prevent disease and ensure wellness, consumers can attain and maintain wellness. Prevention is the wave of the future.... I shouldn't even say the future, it's here. Prevention is the best way to ensure health and to save money, time, effort and prevent pain. The focus needs to be on preventing disease in the first place, and treating disease should be secondary.

Wright

So what resources can you recommend?

Goldie

Well, for instance, resources like *The American Dental Hygienists Association* for oral health information <www.adha.org>. There are many tips for oral health as well as links to other health information. The Smoking Cessation Leadership Center has a website for individuals that would like to stop using tobacco <http://smokingcessationleadership.ucsf.edu/>. Or simply asking questions when you visit your dental hygienist, dentist, physician, nurse, or other health care provider is of value. Reading information is important, whether it is print media or on the Internet. However, that being said, consumers need to make sure that the information they are receiving is from a credible source. Everything found on the Internet is not necessarily the best advice. Make sure that you go to a website of an organization that you feel is credible. Many of the university websites have wonderful information, such as Columbia University, University of Pennsylvania, and others, and places such as the Mayo Clinic, the National Institutes of Health, The American Heart Association, the National Osteoporosis Foundation, the National Women's Health Resource Center, or the Office of Women's

Health websites are other examples. So there are many, many resources that are available to consumers.

Wright

Do you ever recommend products?

Goldie

I do recommend products, and what I do when I recommend or use products is to look at the evidence supporting their claims. There's something now called "evidence based care" in oral health care, and we've borrowed this from medicine where it's been for a long while. Basically, I take my personal experience and combine that with good research to make my recommendations. Not all research is equal, and there are tiers of research and some studies are better than others. I try to choose the best research available when I am deciding which products to recommend. When clients in my office have periodontal infection, I perform procedures such as scaling and root planing (sometimes called debridement) and offer them locally delivered antibiotics, such as Arestin®. www.arestin.com Locally delivered antibiotics have been clinically proven to be more effective than instrumentation alone. So if you are one of the many folks with periodontal infection, ask your dental hygienist or dentist about Arestin® or similar products.

Another example of using evidence to make a decision is...."should I recommend a powered toothbrush rather than a manual toothbrush." I don't only base that recommendation on my personal opinion, I review the studies supporting the claims. And yes, I believe power toothbrushes are an excellent choice for everybody, not just for certain people.

Wright

Why would a power toothbrush be preferable over a manual one?

Goldie

Because some power toothbrushes have been proven to remove more biofilm or plaque, and the bacteria that cause gum disease and tooth decay than manual toothbrushes. They are also gentler than a manual toothbrush!

When you use a manual brush, you can only achieve a two dimensional movement . There is a toothbrush that moves in a three dimensional direction. It is the Oral-B Braun, and it has a three-dimensional movement, where it's not only rotating and oscillating, but it also moves in and out in between the teeth. You could never achieve that movement with your manual toothbrush , and the Cochrane Collaborative has found that toothbrushes that have this rotating, oscillating motion are more effective than manual toothbrushes. Examples are the Oral-B 7000 and the Philips Jordan.

There are certain fluoride rinses that are wonderful not only for children but for adults as well. With proper use, they strengthen the enamel and other parts of the tooth that might be exposed, such as the dentin surfaces when you have gum recession. This is important so that the teeth do not develop tooth decay or sensitivity. These fluoride rinses are very easy to use and very, very effective. Examples are ACT® Fluoride Rinse from Johnson & Johnson or Phos-Flur Rinse® by Colgate. Other times when more oral protection is needed is when someone is undergoing chemotherapy or if they have an eating disorder. They may have dry mouth (xerostomia), and excessive acid because of being sick. Many older adults take many different medications and could have dry mouth, and not be aware of it. There are wonderful products by different companies that can be used to alleviate dry mouth, as that is not a healthy situation. You need saliva to lubricate your mouth in order to chew your food, and saliva has antibacterial and antimicrobial properties, making it a protective agent. Therefore, if you do not have adequate saliva due to chemotherapy or medications, you need to replace that saliva. Many wonderful products can do that. The Biotene® Products from Laclede, Inc. are some of those products, and Gelclair® and Rincinolfrom® the Sunstar Butler Company. Other companies make effective products, as well.

Wright

This has been so interesting. Do you have any further comments or things that you can tell our readers that might help them to be healthier?

Goldie

In a nutshell, be proactive in your health care, and become an advocate for those less fortunate. Make sure that you visit your health care providers on a regular basis, certainly your dental hygienist. He/she is the preventive oral health care specialist and in some cases, can save your life by detecting things like oral cancer or signs of diseases that might be present. So make sure that you see your health care provider and take heed of the messages that they are trying to communicate to you, regarding things that you should be doing at home to not only *attain* but *maintain* oral health and general health.

Wright

Well, I really do appreciate you taking this much time to talk to me today, Maria. It has just really been fascinating.

Goldie

Well, great. Thank you very much yourself.

Wright

Today we have been talking to Maria Perno Goldie, RDH, MS, a noted researcher, author, and speaker. She presents seminars nationally and internationally on topics such as women's health and wellness and periodontal disease, and as we have found this afternoon, she knows a lot about it. And I really appreciate you telling us about it, Maria. Thank you so much!

About The Author

Maria Perno Goldie, RDH, MS brings 30 years of experience to the healthcare arena. As a dental hygienist, speaker, and health advocate, she empowers others to ask questions and become a vital part of their health care. Maria is active at the community level, as well as at an international level. From the speaker's platform, she has addressed national & international groups in an effort to share knowledge and encourage critical thinking. As a passionate dental hygienist, she wants to increase public awareness of who dental hygienists are and what they do. As preventive oral healthcare specialists, dental hygienists can help save lives by detecting oral cancers, oral manifestations of other diseases (such as HIV, eating disorders, or osteoporosis), and referring clients to tobacco cessation programs. Maria is the recipient of the 1999 University of Pennsylvania Dental Hygiene Alumni Achievement Award, and a 2003 winner of the Pfizer/ADHA Award for Excellence in Dental Hygiene.

Maria Perno Goldie, RDH, BA, MS
155 Normandy Court
San Carlos, California 94070
Phone: 650-592-1676
Email: mariaperno1@comcast.net
www.seminarsforwomenshealth.com

Chapter 13

KEVIN SAUNDERS

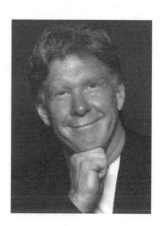

THE INTERVIEW

David E. Wright (Wright)

We're talking to Kevin Saunders. Kevin was born in Downs, Kansas in 1955. He had a wonderful childhood, full of hard work and great love of family, schools, sports, and friends. It was in this environment that he developed the character, courage, and respect for his fellow man that would come to national attention later in his life. A distinguished high school and collegiate athlete, Kevin went to Kansas State University graduating in '78. Upon graduation, Kevin worked as a federal inspector for the USDA. He had a wife, a son, and was truly living the American dream. In 1981, however, it all changed forever. In that year, while working at a Corpus Christi, Texas grain silo complex, a grain dust explosion occurred. Categorized as the worst ever in South Texas history, over ten people were killed. Kevin was blown from a second story building over 300 feet, landing on a concrete parking lot. His body was broken at the chest, severing his spinal cord and paralyzing him from his chest down. With multiple life threatening injuries, Kevin was not expected to live, but live he did. Changing his life and his life's focus, Kevin went on to three Para-Olympics in Seoul, Korea; Barcelona, Spain and Atlanta, Georgia. He was also the first person with a disability ever elected to the

President's Fitness Council by President George H. Bush; and the only member of the council reappointed by President Bill Clinton. In 1990 through 1992, Kevin earned the title of Best All-Around Wheel Chair Athlete in the World. Kevin is currently embarking on his Kevin Saunders Health and Fitness Tour of America. Kevin intends to roll into 125 cities in 50 states over 18 months, spreading his message on health, fitness, using proper exercise and nutrition. Just prior to going to all 50 states Kevin is going to be doing the "BIG PUSH." Kevin is going to push his Quickie wheelchairs from the Canadian border through Detroit, Michigan (who now has the dubious title as America's fattest city) every mile all the way to Laredo, Texas all the way to the Mexican border (this will take approximately 3 months). The prime goal of Kevin's tour is to demonstrate what can be accomplished by anyone regardless of the obstacles we may face in life and to hold a fitness summits with the mayor and key community leaders to discuss the state of the community's health and fitness and facilitate a common sense lasting plan for affecting a grass roots health and fitness commitment. Kevin intends to inspire, motivate, and educate Americans to achieve health and fitness; convey clear, concise messages about exercise and nutrition, and promote and improve wellness for the American workforce and its youth. He will do this through determination and example, just like he has always done it. Kevin, welcome to *Conversations on Health and Wellness*.

Kevin Saunders (Saunders)
Thank you very much. It's an honor to be here.

Wright
Kevin, tell us a little bit about your upcoming tour across America. Man, that thing sounds exciting.

Saunders
First of all, I just want to thank you for the opportunity to tell you about the "Kevin Saunders Health and Fitness Tour of America." I'm really deeply concerned with the health and fitness level of all Americans, and I want to raise awareness of this initiative. There are three reasons why I really am embarking on this tour. Its purpose is to motivate, educate, and inspire all people to achieve health and fitness in America; and secondly, to convey clear, concise and easily understood information about exercise and nutrition; and thirdly, to work with city and community leaders across America by providing resources to

create lasting health and fitness initiatives. I believe lasting success can happen with commitment from individual communities. I want to encourage all community members to get involved in making their community a healthier place to live. The Centers of Disease Control in America show that there's over 300,000 to 400,000 deaths that are related to obesity per year. Sixty-four percent of Americans are overweight and 31 percent of those are considered obese. Our children are considered the world's fattest kids. Being overweight and out of shape puts you at risk for heart disease, cancer, diabetes, and stroke, just to name a few. And these are all important facts that all Americans should be concerned with. The annual direct and indirect health related costs associated with obesity that total over 120 billion dollars a year.

Wright

Wow.

Saunders

I believe that providing clear, easy to understand, free information to remove the confusion is important for all Americans who want to embark on a health and wellness lifestyle. And lastly, I said to work with community leaders to create lasting health and fitness initiatives. The community is where people live, work and play. This is where lasting healthy lifestyle habits are formed and maintained. This goes back to the Centers of Disease Control statistics that show that productivity in America is lost at the tune of 3.9 billion dollars a year due to obesity related illnesses and disease. It's for these reasons that I'm pushing to communities across America from Canada to Mexico the "Big Push" then through key portions of all 50 states with this tour.

Wright

Where will you be starting the tour; where will you be ending it; and how long will it last?

Saunders

Well, Kevin Saunders Health and Fitness Tour has begun on May 5th, which is fitness month. During the month of May we'll be in the state of Texas. And it actually began in Corpus Christi, Texas. This is the city I was injured in the grain elevator explosion, shortly after I graduated from Kansas State University. However, we want to get a

"BIG PUSH" nationally in order to bring national attention to our efforts, So on June 15, 2004, we are doing what we are calling the "BIG PUSH" I am going to push my Quickie wheelchairs from Canada's border through Detroit, Michigan (who now has the dubious title as America's fattest city) all the way to Laredo, Texas, which I will arrive on Labor Day September 6, 2004 (this will take approximately 3 months) across the border into Mexico. Then we will be able to cover all 50 states and adequately cover them in a 14 to 18 month period. We also will be accepting requests and scheduling as many cities as we can in all 50 states while I do the "BIG PUSH." Your requests can be submitted via email to www.HealthandFitnessTour.com in care of Jennifer Martin, our marketing Director. Her email can be found under CONTACTS on the Health and Fitness Tour website.

Wright

Oh, that's great. So why are you doing it?

Saunders

To demonstrate that no matter what obstacles a person may face that they can achieve health and fitness. I'd like to stand up, walk, or even run, but that isn't absolutely necessary for the achievement when it comes to health and fitness. We need to get the clear, concise and easily understood information about health and fitness, set goals and be committed to seeing them through and making health and fitness choices a way of life. If I can do it completely paralyzed from the chest down then anyone can!

Some people may think that I've been dealt a bad hand in my life because I'm paralyzed from the chest down and confined to a wheel chair for life. But I'm doing it because I want to make a difference, be part of the solution to the obesity and overweight out-of-shape epidemic. That's why I set my goals, and made a commitment to push across America and through key portions of all 50 states. Obesity is an epidemic right now, and while there are a lot of reasons for this situation, common sense and proper exercise and nutrition will help get us all on the way to life long health and fitness.

Wright

If you're committed to putting 18 months into this project, what are your expectations of the tour from the standpoint of actually improving people's fitness?

Saunders

To get people motivated, inspired, educated and connected in their local communities and make healthy choices a way of life. We also set our expectation's to have over 95 percent of the American people see or hear about this tour as we go across these 50 states, 125 cities and 180 events. I think that the word of what we are doing to help American get fit on the "BIG PUSH" and the tour will spread and people will start to hear our message across America.

Wright

You know, a lot of people have been screaming about obesity and fitness for many, many years, from the President's council on down. So, tell me, what is different about your message?

Saunders

The difference is two things. One, I'm leading by example. I'm pushing in my Quickie wheelchair into all the cities I'm going through. Two, the Health and Fitness Summits will provide real ways to identify community problems and leave them with real solutions.

The tour is unique because with this summit, the prime goal is to bring a dialogue with myself and the community, with the mayor and key community leaders, to discuss the state of the community's health and fitness. In addition, to facilitate a common sense, long-lasting plan for affecting a grass roots health and fitness commitment. Also, one of the sponsors of the tour is www.ImShapingUp.com, which is the first virtual health and fitness portal website. This website will allow all people regardless of income, race, or ability the access to sound, practical information when it comes to proper exercise, nutrition, rest, stress relief ect. For instance, this gave a us a vehicle to allow Corpus Christi a way to track accountability for exercise and nutrition and to compete against one another as well. So, when the Superintendent of schools made the comment "We're accountable for our fiscal responsibility and our educational responsibility. Why don't we try to be accountable for helping kids with exercise and nutrition?" and they want to take it to the principals, the superintendents of all the different schools said, "Well, we'll challenge your school." The individual school leaders started to challenge one another to see people trying to solve the problem. And this is for everyone; and this will be a competition where everybody wins! We had the answer to help them with the I'mShapingUp.com website.

Wright

Well, you said you were born in 1955, so according to my calculations you're either 49 or close to it.

Saunders

Yes, I'm 48. I was born in December. So at the end of the year I will be 49.

Wright

So, why are you deciding to do this now?

Saunders

Well, I think that now, in my life, with nine years of service to the President's Fitness Council—a combination with George H. Bush and Arnold Schwarzeneger and again under President Bill Clinton as a senior member—I feel that now is a time. Like I said, some people may think I've been dealt a bad hand, but really I feel I'm one of the luckiest people in the world. I've grown because of what's happened to me; and I'm a stronger person mentally and physically.

Wright

Can you tell our readers some of the events that you have planned for the tour?

Saunders

Well, there's some various things that we have that we're going to be doing. There will be races and city proclamations. There will be different openings at hospitals and schools and events that will tie in with the summit meetings to raise awareness in each of these individual communities about the health and fitness summits, the tour and its importance to that individual community.

Wright

I understand the profits are going to three separate organizations. Can you tell us which ones they are; and why did you choose them?

Saunders

Well, we chose the American Heart Association, Diabetes Association and the YMCA's of America. And I believe the American Heart Association and the American Diabetes Association are just two great associations that are trying to help with this obesity epidemic. They do a tremendous amount of things to help the problems that people are encountering across our country that are getting worse due to the growing obesity epidemic. And the YMCA's, they're meant for everybody and they're a great place that's meant for the entire family

Wright

If I was a person reading this book or perhaps listening to this on a radio program somewhere, how would I make a donation to this foundation?

Saunders

First go to our website at www.HealthandFitnessTour.com, click on SPONSORSHIP and you can find multiple ways to help support our message of Health and Fitness for everyone, one community at a time. We welcome individuals and organizations large or small who would like to support our efforts so we can continue to bring our message to communities across America. You can also find out more info under PRESS KIT by clicking on the PDF so you can take a closer look at our message. It will not only give you a lot of great information for the tour, but there is also a page you can print out and send your donations in support of the tour. You can make a donation via credit card as well, just send an e-mail by going to contact on the website letting them know what you would like to do. You can also call the Visibility Company; they are located near Nashville, Tennessee. It's a suburb called Brentwood, Tennessee. Their telephone number is (615) 377-6116; and Jennifer Martin is the person that's in charge of marketing. E-mail Jennifer at jmartin@thevisiblitycompany.com. The name of the actual non-profit is Kevin Saunders Health and Fitness Foundation; and it is non-profit 501-C3 organization. We have a Federal Tax ID number that is 2007149-23.

Wright

So, tell me what motivated you to get into great shape following your accident?

Saunders

I think that the biggest reason was the fact that I got into a real deep depression after my accident. I didn't even know if I wanted to live anymore, but with the help of my friends, I remembered that I did. Exercising and eating right had been a part of my life before my injury. I knew working out and eating right would help get me in a better state of mind. So, it was really a determination to want to regain an active lifestyle and to gain a sense of normalcy back in my life. Since I was paralyzed from the chest down, you can have a tendency to give up when your life and your family and everything falls apart on you. A lot of people look at life when they have tragedy and things like that; and they want to give up. And they don't have a purpose anymore for life. I thought by getting back into shape, I could realize any dreams of being fit and competing again, only this time in a wheelchair. And I could get into competition and wheelchair sporting events.

Wright

So what do you look to for support to keep you on track?

Saunders

Well, most people have specialists that they go to from time to time. They have doctors, lawyers, ect. When it comes to health and fitness, I look to the top fitness trainers and the top registered dieticians and nutritionists because they help me put things in perspective with a common sense approach. They can help me stay healthy and fit for a lifetime. So, they help me stay on track. These people are the experts, the fitness trainers and the registered dieticians and nutritionists, the ones that are good at what they do and trustworthy and they have the best information out there and they want to really help you. That's there goal and they're the ones that can knock you back on that straight line and help you really stay in the best shape of your life. I just wish that everybody had that opportunity; and that's why we're doing this tour to make this information available to everyone. All they've got to do is just get moving, get involved, take part and apply these principles to their lives. There's no doubt if people put these health and fitness principals to use it can change their lives for the better; and I'm really excited about it. I just want to get the word out to people and the communities across America; and I want them to know they can have a better quality of life.

Wright

You talked about taking part in the program. Before we leave, could you tell me how people can find out more about the tour; and when and if you'll be visiting their particular city?

Saunders

You can go to our website at www.HealthandFitnessTour.com; and there you can go to the schedule. It will show you when we'll be in your particular state and what city and the date.

Wright

So its www.HealthandFitnessTour.com?

Saunders

Also, if you want even more precise information on times and things like that, you can call The Visibility Company and speak with Jennifer Martin and that's (615) 377-6116 because most of the time, I'll be out on the road and doing interviews like this via the mobile phone.

Wright

Today, we've been talking to Kevin Saunders. He is taking on the responsibility of inspiring, motivating, and educating Americans to achieve health and fitness by conveying clear, concise messages about exercise and nutrition and to promote and improve wellness for the American workforce and its youth. If you listen to what he just said and if you're reading what he said in the very beginning and you start to just add two figures that he talked about, you'd be in the billions of dollars that we're now wasting on bad health. Kevin, thank you so much for being with us today on *Conversations on Health and Wellness.*

Saunders

Thank you so much for having me. It's been a pleasure.

About The Author

Kevin Saunders, a former Olympic wheelchair athlete named "The Greatest Wheelchair Athlete in the World," and a former member of the President's Council on Physical Fitness and Sports under Presidents George H. Bush and Bill Clinton, is embarking on a revolutionary journey beginning in the Spring 2004 that will change our Nation in very positive ways.

Beginning June 14, 2004, Kevin will begin pushing his wheelchair from Canada to Mexico as a part of his 50-state Health and Fitness Tour of America. Saunders will begin his journey near Canada, in Detroit, Michigan, and will then push his chair nearly 2,000 miles to Laredo, Texas, where he will cross the U.S.-Mexico border. Saunders' mission is to draw attention to the need for communities throughout our nation to focus on lifelong health and fitness for all citizens. In addition to pushing his chair across the country, Saunders will meet with state and local leaders to facilitate a discussion designed to launch a community-based grass-roots approach to achieving a healthier Nation—one community at a time.

Kevin Saunders

C/o Jennifer Martin

The Visibility Company

105 Westpark Drive, Suite 400

Brentwood, Tennessee 37027

Phone: 615-377-6116

Email: jmartin@thevisibilitycompany.com

Chapter 14

DR. NORMAN ROSENTHAL

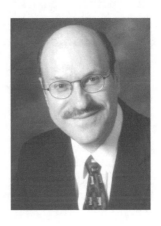

THE INTERVIEW

David E. Wright (Wright)

Today we are talking to Norman Rosenthal. He is best known as the psychiatrist and scientist who first described Seasonal Affective Disorder (SAD) or winter depression and pioneered the use of light in its treatment during his long and distinguished career as a National Institute of Mental Health researcher. For this work he was awarded the prestigious Anna Monica Award and International Prize for Research in Depression. He has conducted extensive research into disorders of mood, sleep, and biological rhythms, which resulted in over 200 scholarly publications. Besides his scholarly writings, Dr. Rosenthal has also written several books for the general public, including *Winter Blues, Seasonal Affective Disorder: What It Is And How To Overcome It,* and *St.-John's-Wort, the Herbal Way To Feeling Good.* Dr. Rosenthal's latest book, *The Emotional Revolution: How the New Science of Feeling Can Transform Your Life.* Dr. Rosenthal's skill at communicating complex scientific material in a way that is both readily understandable and engaging has made him a popular TV and radio guest. He appeared on many national shows including *Good Morning America, CBS Sunday, CBS Morning News, CNN, Fresh Air, All Things Considered, ESPN,* and *The Today Show* just to name a few. Dr. Rosenthal is the medical director of Capital Clinical Research Associates and maintains an active private practice in suburban Maryland. He has been listed among the best doctors in America and in the Guide *to America's Top Psychiatrists*. Dr. Norman Rosenthal, welcome to *Conversations on Health and Wellness*.

Dr. Norman Rosenthal (Rosenthal)
It's good to be here again.

Wright
Dr. Rosenthal, Seasonal Affective Disorder is a fascinating subject. How long have you been engaged in the study of SAD and light therapy?

Rosenthal
A little over 20 years ago, the whole concept of Seasonal Affective Disorder came together for me. I had come from South Africa to the United States, and here much further away from the equator, I felt the seasonal changes in my own mind and in my own body. Then when I saw other people who had similar changes, the pieces of a jigsaw puzzle came together with the help of my colleagues, and we described Seasonal Affective Disorder a condition of regular winter depressions. That was a good 20 years ago.

Wright
You know most of my life I have lived where there were four distinct seasons, and I've always felt differently in each one. I thought it was caused by the memory of events such as swimming in the summer, hiking in the fall, or sledding in the winter. Why do I really feel differently as the seasons change?

Rosenthal
Well, seasons are so rich and so complex, it's hard to pinpoint exactly one thing. I think they provide us with tremendous variety, and I have heard people who have lived in these very tropical areas where the seasons change, and then move to the tropics or closer to the equator and they say they really miss the seasons. They miss the diversity and the richness. So I think we cannot exclude memories, the things that we do at different seasons, the colors, the changing colors, the changing feelings and smells and the sights of the different seasons. But we also need to remember that seasons have a powerful ef-

fect on our biology just like they do on many of the animals that we know about, that we see around us, the squirrels, the bears, the very seasonal animals that breed at different times of the year. We too as humans, although we have thought that we've escaped our environment, remain very locked and have actual changes in our mood, our bodies, our biology and in our brain chemistry in the different seasons.

Wright

You have said that the pain of depression, anxiety, and other emotional disturbances is as real as physical pain. It deserves to be understood, studied, treated, healed, and reimbursed by insurance just like the pain of any other illness. I know your pioneering work in the field of SAD and life therapy has helped in the identification and the treatment of seasonal depression in people, but do the insurance companies recognize these advances and do they cover them?

Rosenthal

You know this is the sad fact of American life. Of course, firstly, there are so very many people who don't have medical insurance at all. But even amongst those who do, there is a double standard whereby so called physical illnesses get properly reimbursed or reimbursed at a higher rate and mental illnesses get reimbursed at a very low rate, and that's one of the sad facts. Members of Congress and the Senate have tried to turn it around, but so far have been unsuccessful. But certainly, as a psychiatrist who sees the pain that conditions like depression or schizophrenia cause human beings and it seems just plain wrong not to reimburse them at comparable rates to other kinds of illnesses.

Wright

Someone had told me in an interview a few months ago that the pharmaceutical industry financed almost everything in the medical community. That shouldn't make any difference, should it? I mean, the pharmaceutical companies would come into play with medicine for anxiety and that sort of thing just as much as a pain of ulcers, wouldn't they?

Rosenthal

Indeed, the pharmaceutical companies are a huge power in developing new forms of treatment, and I think we are quite indebted to them for coming up with many novel medications. Of course, Prozac and Zoloft, just to name two, have been huge best sellers with many others as well. I won't list them all. But these, of course, come out of research that is funded by the pharmaceutical companies. So I think that they have a lot to offer. To some degree the pharmaceutical companies all stay powerful, however, and that should be balanced against government funding of research, which is also very important.

Wright

One of your clients has written and I would like to quote here, "For years my mood energy dropped with the leaves, and I felt ashamed and saddened by my inability to control my winter depression. Dr. Rosenthal's book, *Winter Blues*, gave me the tools to effectively treat SAD. Now my winters are productive and happy." What tools do you give your readers in your book, *Winter Blues*?

Rosenthal

The first tool I try to give my readers is just self-awareness to understand how their moods are changing with the changing seasons. I think insight and knowledge is power when it comes to the brain as in other aspects of life. Once they know what they are suffering from in the case of winter depression, they can plan, they can prepare, and they can use some of the techniques that have been found helpful like increasing their environmental light, like exercise, like stress management and dietary control, and in some people medications may also be extremely helpful.

Wright

You've been internationally recognized for your work in depression research and you are listed as one of the best doctors in America and in The *Guide to America's Top Psychiatrists*. How prevalent is depression in the United States? How does it negatively affect our lives?

Rosenthal

They estimate that about 17 million people suffer from depression, which is really a huge number.

Wright

Seventeen million?

Rosenthal

Yes, it's a huge number and there's also evidence that depression is occurring more and more in younger people, which of course takes a huge toll on the country in so many ways. Just to quantify the cost of depression to the society, they reckon it's 43 billion dollars per year both in terms of the cost of treatment; but also in terms of lost productivity, absenteeism, or what they've called presenteeism, which means a person is there at work but is really unable to be properly engaged in productive efforts.

Wright

Is it caused by stress?

Rosenthal

Stress can certainly bring it on. Loss can bring it on. There's also evidence of the genetic basis, and I think a lack of community and a lack of good things in a person's life can do it. So many things can bring on depression. In the case of winter depression, the lack of light can do it. So there are many ways whereby somebody can become depressed.

Wright

Why do you think that it is beginning to affect people at a younger age?

Rosenthal

They really don't know. One thing that's been raised as a possibility is drug use. Certainly drugs can induce depression. People have suggested perhaps that the young people are less connected with their families and their communities which are protective influences perhaps in the development of depression.

Wright

Yeah, I cannot remember a time when I was a young boy that I did not eat meals with my family, I'm 64 years old now and I have a 14 year old, and most of the time we do not eat together.

Rosenthal

Well, I think that really does say something, doesn't it?

Wright

It gives me something to think about, I'll tell you. Let's talk about light therapy. First of all, what is light therapy? How does light affect us?

Rosenthal

Well, of course, we've known for centuries that light is critical for enabling us to see. What's really quite new over the last couple of decades is the idea that light has important biological effects on us over and above enabling us to see. One of these effects seems to be to maintain our mood and energy level, and that's why when light levels decline in the fall and in the winter months, some people who are sensitive to this lose energy and have a decline in their mood. Light therapy is simply an attempt to replace the missing light. This is done by means of special light fixtures which are boxes with fluorescent tubes filtered by a plastic diffusing screen that have been shown in research studies to be highly effective in reversing the symptoms of winter depression.

Wright

Are the same bulbs used as the fluorescent bulbs used that we can go down to our friendly Wal-Mart store and pick up, or is it special light?

Rosenthal

The tubes themselves can be regular off the shelf tubes. The trick, however, is to have a lot of light packed into one place, because it seems that the amount of light is very important. Also the timing of light can be very important, and light treatment in the morning seems to be the most effective type of treatment for most people.

Wright

I found a few places on the internet that sell light boxes, which I didn't know what they were, or Dawn's Simulators, I think they called them. Are these the tools that you recommend, and do they work for everyone suffering from SAD.

Rosenthal

Yes, indeed those are some companies that put out light boxes. I have listed on my website, which in case your listeners or readers would like to know about is www.normanrosenthal.com, I have listed a link to the light box companies that have been around for many years whose products follow certain guidelines and who stand behind their work. For people with SAD they can be extremely helpful, but you know nothing works for everybody. That's why it's always good to have some tricks up your sleeve. So for some people the lights may be somewhat helpful, but not do the entire job. Those people may require medications as well as light therapy. For other people, they may be a nuisance to have to use, and for those people it's also a comfort to know that other treatments are available.

Wright

Would it also help to be out of doors more often early in the morning when there is light rather than staying in the house?

Rosenthal

Definitely. I recommend people go for morning walks. I follow my own advice. I feel that it's a very good thing to combine aerobic exercise with exposure to light, and also walking around the neighborhood. If it is a safe neighborhood it is another way of linking yourself to the community and having that combination of social contact with light and exercise, combining all these healthy and pleasurable influences together.

Wright

Many people around the world became acquainted with you because of your study of the herb St. John's Wort and it's effect on emotional health. For those of us who don't know much about this herbal remedy, will you tell us a little bit about your findings?

Rosenthal

Yes. It's intriguing to think that the extract of a plant can actually improve our mood, but in fact St. John's Wort is really the oldest documented antidepressant around. There is an Italian chemist named Angelo Solla, who 350 years ago carefully documented how he would give the extract of St. John's Wort to melancholic people, people who suffered from depression and how it seemed to be specifically helpful to depressed people. Then in Germany, in the early part of the 20th century, research in St. John's Wort resurged and a lot of research was done. By now there are many, many studies that show an effect of St. John's Wort, so it is an active antidepressant and should be considered as one of many options for people suffering from depression.

Wright

When it comes to herbal remedies and treatments, there seems to be two camps. Some people are completely open minded about the positive effect of certain actual treatments and give credible personal testimony. Others seem to be completely close minded. Is there a correlation in the scientific community to a person's predisposition about the effective of herbal medicine and the actual clinical effectiveness?

Rosenthal

Remember that the idea of medications coming from herbs is nothing new. Digitalis came from a Foxglove, and an anticancer drug came from the plant Little Periwinkle. So the idea that plants are sources of potent medications is not a new thing. I guess that one factor at work here is that there was an act passed by which herbs and dietary supplements are not regulated like medications. What that really means is that it's hard to know what you are getting when you get herbal extracts because they are not standardized. So they don't conform to the usual standards. They don't always have as much herb in them as they say, and also because they are not easily patentable. There isn't the commercial incentive to study them as rigorously. So those are the problems in terms of knowing exactly what's what with herbs. But by the same token that they probably have got tremendous value in some instances. As I said, St. John's Wort is healthful with mood.

Kava kava is an herb that's healthful for anxiety, although recently there have been some reports of liver damage with that herb, you see, which justifiably scares people away from it. But here again, if it was a pharmaceutical product, the company would swoop in and figure out how to prevent any damage and produce a safe product. Now since it is not a regulated product, there's a sort of halo of discomfort that surrounds it because of this liver damage.

Valerian for sleep, so many herbs can affect the mind in positive ways. It's just that you're not quite sure what you are getting with the preparations.

Wright

I take Saw palmetto, but I am not sure if it is an herb or what.

Rosenthal

It's an herb for prostates.

Wright

Yes. I take that religiously at least twice a day, and also I read an article just a few days ago that another thing that helps enlarged prostate is pumpkin seeds. It said go to your health store to find them. I went to the health store and, of course, they didn't have it. The Saw palmetto helped considerably and if anything else would help, I would certainly be opened to taking it.

Rosenthal

Well no, there's certainly data in relation to Saw palmetto. I don't know about the pumpkin seed.

Wright

In the last decade, I've notice more and more breakthroughs in medical research that contradicts long standing beliefs about health and medicine. I'm certain that you've been a part of some of this research. How can I, an average person with limited understanding of these things, know what is real and what is snake oil?

Rosenthal

I still believe that science is a critical method for separating the real from the illusory. I think that we should go with things that are scientifically backed. That having been said, sometimes the science just isn't there and we still may need to go with our own experience or the experience of those we respect in deciding how best to lead our lives.

Wright

Dr. Rosenthal, do you have an overriding personal philosophy of health that you could share with our readers?

Rosenthal

Yes. I believe that we need to keep in line our intellectual mind, our emotional mind, and our body. These are the three domains that we need to take care of, and that if we take care of all those, we have the best chance not only of leading long lives, but of leading good and healthy ones as well.

Wright

Before we close, could you tell us what is on the horizon for Dr. Norman Rosenthal?

Rosenthal

Well, I would follow up on what I think leads to a healthy life by sort of off-lining how I personally am going to try to pursue that. In terms of physical health, I exercise regularly. I have started Yoga, which is a wonderful. It is different from a western way of thinking. It emphasizes relaxation and stretching and moment-to-moment consciousness of being, which I think are tremendously valuable. So I am careful with exercise, with Yoga, with diet, and of course with regular checkups with my own physician, all the ordinary things that western medicine can give us now. For example, we've now learned that lowering cholesterol is very valuable, and that the drugs that do it can have all sorts of unexpected payoffs. That's the physical piece. The emotional piece, I feel it's very important to identify the meaningful people in one's life and keep in touch with them, and have a constructive to and fro. If there are people who are important to you that you really care about, but there's been a falling out, I think if you can mend your fences, that's a good thing. I think it's so unhealthy to carry anger and negative feelings about with you if you don't have to. You should dwell in a positive zone, these are things that I personally try and follow. I think they are not any good for our bodies, they're good for our souls.

But I also for myself love an adventure, and writing those books has been a huge adventure to me. But now, I've embarked upon an adventure that is both new and old. I am back to doing research, basically testing new medications in various psychiatric illnesses and also eager to continue to study the effects of our physical environment on our brains and our bodies. It's an intriguing thing to me, and I had left research for three or four years. Now that I am back in it again, I feel like a Labrador that's been let loose in the water. It's so much fun, and I am eager to both discover and contribute at the same time. These are some of the things that I hope to have in store for me.

Wright

Well, that's good news for those of us who will be recipients of that work, I can assure you. I certainly appreciate all the time that you have taken with me today, Dr. Rosenthal. It's always a pleasure to talk to you. Before the interview started I told my wife I had an interview to do. She said, "Who are you going to speak to?" And I said, "Dr. Norman Rosenthal." She says, "Uh oh! He is one of your favorites. You respect him as much as anybody." And she's right about that.

Rosenthal

Well, I think you and I have a mutual admiration society because I remember after our last conversation feeling quite elated for hours afterwards because you are so enlivening and so positive. One ends up feeling so good having spoken to you. Are you sure you aren't a therapist in a pre-existing incarnation?

Wright

That could be!

Rosenthal

Any time, any time. I look forward to continuing the conversations over the years.

Wright

Thank you so much for being with us Dr. Rosenthal. Today we've been talking to Dr. Norman Rosenthal, who is best known, of course, as a psychiatrist. As we have learned today, he is quite knowledgeable on that and other topics as well. Thank you so much, Dr. Rosenthal.

Rosenthal

Have a good day.

About The Author

Through his research, writings, speaking engagements and private practice, Dr. Norman Rosenthal has been the voice of hope for those suffering from depression and emotional distress. His pioneering work in the field of Season Affective Disorder (SAD) and photo therapy created a revolution in the identification and treatment of seasonal depression.

Dr. Norman Rosenthal

www.normanrosenthal.com

Chapter 15

JENNY HERRICK

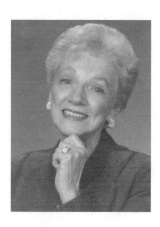

THE INTERVIEW

David E. Wright (Wright)

We are talking to Jenny Herrick. Jenny is a recognized leader in the field of humor and health. She travels throughout the country teaching her audiences how to lighten up. As a motivational humorist, she shares a powerful message about the enormous power of humor. Her clients are from health care facilities, professional organizations and businesses throughout the United States. With over thirty five years of professional experience, here is a lady who wears many hats: nurse, dog handler (yes, that's right), advocate for teens, professional speaker, humor therapist, clown ambassador, work place cheerleader, mother, grandmother, sister, friend and community advocate. She's a graduate of the Lutheran School of Nursing, in Sioux City, Iowa, a looooong time ago (these are her words). She received a Bachelor of Applied Science with a major in Psychology from Westmar University, LeMars, Iowa. She received her training as a clown from the University of Wisconsin Clown College in LaCrosse, Wisconsin and her Laughter Leadership Training in Columbus, Ohio. She has traveled internationally as a clown with the famous clown/physician, Dr. Patch Adams, and again as a clown to Ground Zero to spread "mirth aid" to the rescue workers in 2001. She is a member of the National Speakers Association, Applied Association for Therapeutic Humor, National Association for Self-Esteem, The Fellowship of Merry Christians and Clowns of American International. In 2002, she was nominated for the Woman of Excellence award, in the Striving to Make a Difference category. Ms. Herrick, welcome to *Conversations on Health and Wellness.*

Jenny Herrick (Herrick)
Thank you, David, for having me.

Wright
Is it true that laughter really is the best medicine and if so what are the benefits?

Herrick
The benefits are somewhat debatable, but laughter is definitely considered the best medicine. There are many good reasons for this. First of all, it's a gift which means it's something you can give and receive. You don't need a prescription for it or a membership to a health club. A good hearty belly laugh will give you the very same type of a "runner's high" as you would get from running the marathon! Another great benefit is you don't need to worry about overdosing.

Wright
So I imagine this type of medicine is available to everyone?

Herrick
Of course it is, however some people aren't aware of that, which is sad. People don't utilize this gift, not realizing how valuable, powerful and beneficial laughter can be. So that's where I come in as a motivational humorist.

Wright
I've learned there's something considerably new developing in the United States, called the World Laughter Tour, whose ultimate purpose is to achieve peace one laugh at a time. Are you involved in that purpose, and can others become involved?

Herrick

Indeed I am! I'm a strong advocate of the World Laughter Tour . . . it's philosophy and purpose. This is something I strongly believe in and continue to inform and promote to my audiences wherever I go. I'm very proud to say at this time that I happen to be the only Certified Laughter Leader in the state of Iowa. In order to become a Certified Laughter Leader, a person is trained in eleven hours of intense theory and practice. You are taught how to lead people in what's called unstructured laughter. In other words, it's a known fact, that people think we have to have something funny in order to make them laugh, but as certified laughter leaders we teach people that's NOT necessary. We CAN laugh without a purpose, simply because the end result is so beneficial and therapeutic.

Wright

Your background as a former nurse, animal welfare activist, educator, consultant, traveling clown, and not to forget your present profession, a professional speaker, has brought about a change in your attitude regarding quality of life. Could you explain how this came about and perhaps why?

Herrick

Yes, I'd love to! My attitude towards life has changed a lot during my lifetime. I think everyone experiences circumstances that are not so full of joy and cheer and most of us have what we refer to as our "crosses to bear." It just so happens that my cross to bear occurred quite early in my life, in fact at age twenty-seven, I became a widow, was left with two tiny boys to raise alone . . . something like that makes a person grow up in a hurry. Thank God for my nursing degree and my spiritual faith, I was able to carry on. After nine years I remarried and once again experienced joy becoming a mother to a baby girl at age 39. I live each day to the fullest because I have learned how fragile life really is and should not be taken for granted. I started my speaking career 15 years ago and have found out how gratifying that can be. It's not uncommon to have an audience member come up to me after a presentation, give me a hug and say, "Oh, how I needed to hear that." Or others have come up with tears in their eyes thanking me for giving them permission to laugh again. Sometimes it's been "My boss should hear your message." My topics all pertain to laughter and how to have joy in our lives, how to have a more fun-filled and laughter filled life. We all have the "ups and downs" in our lives.

Wright

Your philosophy of life...you say, it's meant to be lived. Isn't everybody who is breathing living? Is it possible to develop this belief?

Herrick

Yes, I'm so glad you asked that. Is everyone who is breathing, living? No, no, no, a hundred times NO...there are people who are NOT really living. I believe in order to live life to the fullest; a person needs to have a strong faith in the Lord and welcome each day with a smile on your face and joy in your heart. This is something we all have to work at...it just doesn't come and hit you like a bolt of lightning. You need to open your eyes, take a deep breath and put on your comic glasses. It comes from looking around and finding the joy, the silliness and playfulness in our lives. You've heard those good old familiar sayings..."you've got to take time to smell the coffee," or "put your rose colored glasses on." Actually, all that means is to be receptive to what life has to offer us! I proclaim to be a humor "expert" and consequently am known as a lady who "walks the talk," which means I integrate humor into my very being on a daily basis.

Wright

Do you feel that attitude is something that is simultaneous with a sense of humor?

Herrick

Our sense of humor depends entirely on our attitude. So, just what IS a sense of humor? The word "humor" comes from the Latin word "umor," which means to be flexible, to flow, like water . . . to go with the flow. If you ask a group of individuals . . . what is a sense of humor . . . oftentimes they don't even know if they have one or not. All it is, is ATTITUDE! Attitude is everything!

Wright

How important do you think it is to take risks?

Herrick

The older I get the more risks I take! What have I got to lose? You're going to gain every time you take a risk. Sometimes it may not always be for the better, but how are you going to know if you don't take a risk?

Wright

Is there a difference what you have found in therapeutic humor and in laughter?

Herrick

Yes, as hospital clown therapist I consider all clowning in health care facilities, whether it's a nursing home, a retirement home, hospice or hospital that these are the type of places where humor therapy is definitely needed and is lacking most of the time. If people would just be open to finding the "funny" in their world and daily lives, such as when standing in the checkout line at the grocery store. Instead of becoming uptight and frustrated, glancing at your watches and letting out big sighs, talk to the other people in the line. Sometimes I even talk to the magazines and candy rack! (That's a different type of humor, but it can and does relieve frustration and stress.) So again, the therapy comes into play because it has been proven through studies that we can't be full of stress and tension at the same time we are thinking positive thoughts! Isn't that neat?

Wright

Absolutely

Herrick

Just by putting a smile on our face, we not only look better but we are relieving our stress.

Wright

My mother was in a nursing home for a period of time and I noticed there was a program in which there was a clown ministry and another program in which there was a dog who was trained to visit the people, even the ones who were seriously demented. These residents came "out of their shell" whenever the clowns and the dog came to visit. What's that all about?

Herrick

That's true therapy. Those examples are just a couple of many. There's pet therapy, music therapy, touch therapy and now humor therapy!

Wright

I noticed that a lady who played the piano. She played old familiar songs and hymns. There were people who had not said a word in who knows how long remembering the words to the songs.

Herrick

Isn't that wonderful?

Wright

So when you think of connection, what comes to your mind?

Herrick

Connection! We all need connection in our daily lives. We all need to feel connected to someone or something! Without connection, I think it's probably like a bird who has lost its ability to fly, it's floundering...no direction or purpose. What a shame when we, as individuals, encounter this dilemma. I believe there's magic in connection. When we laugh WITH people, sharing a joke, a story, a special look at a special person in our lives, that's what I think of when I think of connectiveness. How vitally profound and important that is.

Wright

So how much research have you done, both in theory and practice regarding what humor does and can do to help us be healthier and happier individuals?

Herrick

David, I've probably devoted the past fifteen years of my life to learning all I can about humor and it's benefits. I've put in a lot of time and effort into my own personal research by turning off the TV, not finding the time to read a good juicy book for years, avoided long non-productive telephone conversations and gearing my research towards almost entirely that of humor, laughter and comic relief and what it can do to us physiologically and psychologically. Research is continually being done in universities. When I started my own quest to learn what has been proven, humor and health were just not simultaneous...not anything you associated with each other. It wasn't until the early 1980s that humor and medicine were introduced and used together in the field of medicine. Research is ongoing and probably always will be. I, myself, don't need proof that laughter works. I say, "Use it... or lose it...your funny bone, that is!"

Wright

Recently I interviewed Dr, Bernie Siegel, who has really done some outstanding research on the subject. I remember when my wife was going through cancer, it kind of turned our family upside down for a couple years and I remember some of those books, Dr. Siegel wrote that were very helpful. What do you see for the future regarding pain reduction, via the use of humor?

Herrick

Being familiar with Dr. Siegel's work and also that of Norman Cousin, I believe that humor can be a developed skill. There are people who are "humor impaired" and there's a solution to this problem. There are ways to help people find it, see it and utilize it. Paul McGhee has developed a program in which he teaches humor skills and how to use it to our benefit. With the release of endorphins and psychoimmunology (PNI), our bodies tend to have their own "inner pharmacy" and pain reduction is very possible through the use of laughter. Dr. Patch Adams travels the world with a delegation of clowns to spread this very theory. The World Laughter Tour is teaching this very skill through the formation off laughter clubs solely for the purpose that people CAN laugh, SHOULD laugh and NEED to laugh in order to achieve everything better in themselves and the world.

Wright

So, do you believe that there really are humor impaired individuals?

Herrick

Yes, I do...have even known some personally!

Wright

Is there any hope for them?

Herrick

There is, as long as they have an open mind and are receptive to learning the skills. I've encountered individuals in my audiences that sit with their arms folded across their chest, a scowl on their face and a look that says, "Go ahead, I dare you to just try and make me laugh... "That's a challenge for me, but more often than not when that hour is up, these are the individuals who come up and admit that was the most fun they've had in a long time...that they hadn't laughed so much for a long time.

Wright

Do you feel that these individuals who laugh often are more healthy and hearty and live longer than those who don't laugh as much?

Herrick

I believe that and am very seldom sick myself. My attitude is "life is too short to be taken too seriously." I proclaim to be a "life enthusiast!" My belief is that we find our own happiness. It's OUR choice whether we're going to have a GOOD day or not and why waste a moment whining or complaining.

Wright

You know it occurred to me that people in the medical field like Dr. Siegel and Patch Adams, whose life was portrayed in the movie by Robin Williams are living what they preach and subsequently are probably healthier because of that. They see a lot of people suffering and dying and that sort of thing; children with serious illnesses. It seems to me that it should work both ways, on the laugher and the laughee.

Herrick

I've never heard that expression, but I like it!

Wright

I just made it up!

Herrick

Good for you! It's catchy, isn't it? Patch Adams is a phenomenal man and after traveling with him (as a clown) for twelve days to another country, it changed my life. I am unable to resist talking to total strangers and have learned there are very few limits to finding the humor and joy in life. Patch has a philosophy that in order to get to the bottom of a patient's problem (illness) it's necessary to find out what kind of a sense of humor they have; what it takes to make them laugh. So he might spend two hours or two months to do just that and then he says, "Let's do it!" That's one of the problems with people today. They are waaaaay too serious, too uptight, too afraid to take risks, afraid they will be humiliated and that people might laugh AT them. Wouldn't it be fun if we would "grow down" instead of growing up. To be a child again, to be child-like, not childish. Let's go back to chewing bubble gum and blowing big huge bubbles and letting them burst all over our faces, into our hair and playing jacks and hop-scotch, kick the can (what does THAT say about my age?).

Wright

Oh, yes! I'm probably older than you are!

Herrick

Oh, get out of town! Nobody is OLDER than I am!

Wright

I had a sixty fifth birthday last month!

Herrick

Oh, you're getting up there, boy! Just turned seventy myself!

Wright

Oh, my!

Herrick

Oh my! You didn't have to say THAT, David. I can still outwork a lot of forty year old women and maybe even a man or two!

Wright

Sounds like it!

Herrick

Well, yes, I do believe that if you have a wonderful sense of humor, a wonderful joy of living and a positive attitude, you're going to be less sick and subsequently may live longer!

Wright

Let me ask you a final question.

Herrick

Sure

Wright

I know you are probably someone who sets goals and you sound like you have plans and dreams that you still have to accomplish. What's in the cards for the next few years for Jenny Herrick?

Herrick

Oh, bless you. Yes, I am a goal setter from the word, "Go!" Whenever I've set a goal, I've achieved it! I'm not able to tell you right today, what my next goal is, other than to complete this chapter for our new book. I'm going to continue to practice my philosophy: Enjoy life to the fullest (perhaps with a new love in my life). That's all I'm going to share with you, David. What do you think?

Wright

I think that's great! I've always wanted to be, when I see all my friends dying and everything . . .I would like to be shot when I'm ninety by an irate husband!

Herrick

Oh, how cute!

Wright

Innocently, of course!

Herrick

Of course! By mistake! I guess my final goal is to have a "standing ovation" up yonder!

Wright

Well, that WOULD be a great thing and maybe for all of us, but when you put it that way, I believe that would be a great goal for me as well.

Herrick

As a former dog trainer, I used to say, "When I die, I hope it's with a good dog at the end of my leash!" Now I've changed that to having my last standing ovation!

Wright

I really appreciate that time you've taken with me today. I've learned a lot. It's been fun and I wish you every success in the world as you reach your goals.

Herrick

Thank you, David, you're very sweet.

Wright

Today, we've been talking with Jenny Herrick, on *Conversations on Health and Wellness*. She's a recognized leader in the field of humor and travels all over the country teaching people how to "lighten up!" She's had thirty-five years professional experience and I really appreciate the time you've taken with us today.

Herrick

Thank YOU, David

About The Author

Jenny Herrick is a gifted speaker filled with a contagious enthusiasm for living. Jenny Herrick has an exciting style of communication from the platform as she shares her personal reasons why we should "lighten up!"

She is a member of the Applied Association for Therapeutic Humor, the Fellowship of Merry Christians, Toastmaster's International, International Clowns of America and National Speakers Association. She's a college clown graduate who utilizes her fun-loving skills to bring joy and humor to individuals in healthcare facilities not only in this country but overseas, as well. She's had the unique experience of traveling to China with a Fun Medicine delegation led by the famous clown/physician, Dr. Patch Adams in 2000. In 2001, she joined other clown ambassadors in New York City to provide 'mirth aid' to rescue workers at Ground Zero which she says consequently "changed my life."

Jenny's personal experiences have provided her with stories to pique your interest about many aspects of the humorous side of life. Her depth of knowledge, sense of humor and caring attitude leave her audiences inspired and motivated to not "sweat the small stuff!"

Here's a lady who believes the quality of your attitude determines the quality of your relationships, not to mention just about everything else in your life.

Jenny Herrick
Motivational Humorist
ALL KIDDING ASIDE
2829 So. Cypress
Sioux City, Iowa 51106
Phone: 712-276-4315
Email: Bestma34@Cableone.net
www.allkiddingaside.biz

Chapter 16

DR. SHERENE MCHENRY, LPC

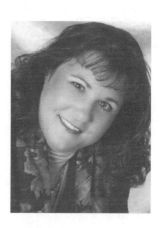

THE INTERVIEW

THE INTERVIEW

David E. Wright (Wright)

Today, we're talking to Dr. Sherene McHenry. As an expert in human relations, Dr. Sherene McHenry is an accomplished author, international speaker and consultant who specializes in helping organizations, couples and individuals create and sustain environments that generate exceptional motivation and success. She is a graduate professor at Central Michigan University, a Licensed Professional Counselor, and a member of the National Speakers Association. Sherene has authored a college text and multiple journal articles, and is currently writing a series of books focusing on improving relationships. With her dynamic personality and strong sense of humor, Dr. McHenry has informed and delighted a wide range of audiences around the world. Dr. McHenry, welcome to *Conversations on Health and Wellness*.

Sherene McHenry (McHenry)

Thank you, I'm happy to be here.

Wright

Why do you think people are particularly interested, even anxious, about health and wellness issues these days?

McHenry

We live in tumultuous times. Our world changed drastically on 9-11 and we now question our individual and collective well-being and safety. Further challenging our illusion of control, the economy is shaky, and layoffs, downsizing and unemployment are on the rise. We also live in a 24-7-365 news culture where we are inundated with graphic and distressing images, bad news, and lots of hype. All this can lead to a great deal of stress and anxiety.

Wright

Life as we've known it is changing at an increasingly alarming rate; and the increase in violent and uncontrollable acts is undeniable. How can individuals stay grounded in an ever-changing, increasingly frightening world?

McHenry

If we want to stay grounded, we must focus on what is under our control. Individually, we can do little about the economy, terrorism and what's going on around the world. However, we have a great deal of control over our personal choices and where we focus our energies. Realizing there's a difference between what we can and cannot control allows us to expend our energy and resources strategically. While we may still get tossed about by the storms of life, focusing on the seven pillars of healthy living provides an anchor that will hold.

Wright

You identify the need for individuals to develop authenticity and congruence. Those aren't terms we hear very frequently. What makes them central to an individual's overall wellness and health; and how does one go about becoming authentic and congruent?

McHenry

Being authentic and congruent is being honest with ourselves and with others about whom we are, what we think and how we feel. While not a license to say everything that comes into our head, authenticity and congruence constitute knowing who we are, what's important to us and interacting honestly with others. Until we develop a strong sense of authenticity and congruence, we're like chameleons ever changing to meet the desires of others. Once we develop a sense of authenticity and congruence, we become anchored and no longer need to live at the whim of what's going on around us. Individuals can do a number of things to develop authenticity and congruence. The first is simply being real. I used to believe I needed to be perfect in order for others to like and respect me. What I've learned is that perfection doesn't attract others. People are drawn to individuals who are real, imperfections and all. A gift I regularly give is letting others know my faults and mishaps. For example, when the first couple I ever counseled told me they were experiencing sexual problems, I got so nervous I started to giggle. That's not real empathic for a trained counselor! When I share experiences like this, others see that I'm human and learn that it's ok for them to make mistakes as well.

In order to be authentic and congruent; it's important to know who we are including our likes, dislikes, personality preferences and love languages. We also need to move beyond thinking that everyone else is, or should be, just like us. Individuals are unique; and developing a sense of authenticity and congruence allows us to understand, accommodate and work together instead of against each other. I could go on about this forever, but the last point I'll make is that most of us regularly send mixed messages where our words don't match up with our body language or voice tone. Unfortunately, when this happens, people either don't believe us or disregard what we're saying! For example, when people who are angry share their frustrations with a smile, they are regularly discounted which results in their becoming even more upset. If individuals want to be heard, believed and taken seriously, their facial expressions, voice tone and body language must match their words and feelings. Once these factors line up, individuals are taken far more seriously in all facets of life.

Wright

It's very frustrating. I've thought many times that everybody on Earth should be given an Academy Award simply for masking. It's hard. When I'm hiring people, the message I get is often miles apart from the one I get later.

McHenry

I fully agree! Having a background in careers, I know the responses employers like to hear. However, I chose to authentically and congruently answer each question because I'm unwilling to set myself up for the frustration of not being able to be myself. Furthermore, I don't want someone to hire me and then be angry and disappointed because I am different than how I presented myself. My belief is, "If you want to hire me great; if you don't, that's ok." Being authentic and congruent allows me to: 1). Judge if there's a good fit; 2). Be myself once I'm hired; and, 3). Allows others to know what they're getting. It's a gift that goes both ways. It's not always easy, but well worth it in the long run.

Wright

I agree! Sherene, you've also identified the ability to develop and set appropriate boundaries as being key to enjoying wellness and good health. To many, the term "boundaries" sounds punitive and unattractive. Just what is a boundary; and who needs them anyway?

McHenry

A boundary is simply a screening mechanism. Healthy boundaries are tight enough to screen out what's bad, or that for which there isn't sufficient time or resources. Simultaneously, healthy boundaries are porous enough to let in that which is good. Organizations and individuals with weak boundaries allow others to take advantage of, or harm, them financially, physically, emotionally, and/or spiritually. Additionally, they over commit themselves and their resources, significantly reducing their chances for success. On the other end of the spectrum are those with rigid boundaries who screen most everything, and everyone, out. While they may be fairly successful at keeping out the bad, by failing to let in what's good, they also end up isolated and missing opportunities. There's a balance point between the two extremes that must be continually checked and maintained. Even those with good boundaries occasionally miss an opportunity and/or let something negative slip in "under their radar." When this occurs, those with good boundaries readjust to ensure that it doesn't happen again.

Wright

The term boundaries has a negative connotation. It simply does, but you're not talking about setting boundaries on others; you're talking about setting your own boundaries for yourself, which is positive.

McHenry

Healthy boundaries are positive because they allow organizations, couples and individuals to judiciously use their time, talent and resources. However, when boundaries are violated, such as employees coming to work late, a response must be determined. "Bad" behavior left unchecked, rarely goes away and almost always worsens. For example, when employers don't address tardiness, three things happen: 1). Those who are late, learn its ok to be so; 2). Over time they push the boundary further and come in even later; and, 3). Those who are on time become increasingly resentful. Therefore, consequences aren't set to be punitive, but to help the person as well as the organization. It's imperative to understand that setting boundaries is particularly difficult in the beginning, and that resistance and a period of testing must be expected. The good news is that poor behaviors can be eradicated with consistently enforced boundaries. There are other benefits to setting and holding appropriate boundaries. Those who set boundaries don't have to make excuses or overlook inappropriate behavior, therefore, their frustration doesn't mount to the point that they end up "losing it" over small infractions. In fact, individuals who deal with problems as they occur rarely lose their temper.

I think it's helpful to also look at boundaries from a parenting point of view. Continuing the "being late" example, most parents worry that something terrible may have happened to their child once curfew passes. If parents want their children home on time, they simply need to state, and enforce boundaries.

For example, "Your curfew was 12:00 am, and when you weren't home on time I began to worry. You've lost the privilege of going out next weekend." Parents who set and hold boundaries have children who are respectful. While the next weekend might not be much fun for the parents or the child, children who know there will always be an unpleasant consequence, come home on time. When it comes to setting boundaries, organizations and individuals tend to fall into one of three camps. Healthy ones consistently set and enforce appropriate boundaries that aren't punitive. Their attitude is primarily, "Here's what I can live with; here's what I can't. If that works for you, great. If it doesn't, that's okay. But I'm going to make choices based on the boundaries that have been set." Then there are those who continually over-function for others, as well as, those who regularly under-function by asking others to make exceptions or to do more than their share. In our society, it is extremely common to see individuals over-functioning and therefore enabling others to under-function. Parents do homework for their children. A coworker or boss picks up the slack for a colleague who regularly under-functions. Unfortunately, over-functioning isn't helpful in the long run as it results in those who under-function failing to develop the skills and behaviors necessary for living a happy, healthy and productive life. Furthermore, rarely having to face the consequences of their actions stunts the self regulation necessary for individuals to mature into responsible adults capable of having stellar careers and fulfilling relationships. My hope is that people will begin to see boundaries not as a punitive and negative, but as protective and enhancing!

Wright

You didn't read my life story before this interview, did you?

McHenry

I didn't.

Wright

Well, I'm listening to my life, especially about the children. I've done everything you've said both bad and good. I recognize what you're saying. It's very difficult.

McHenry

Boundaries are difficult and a lifelong process. Setting and holding boundaries protects and grows the organization, couple, individual and especially children.

Wright

You also talk about the need for cultivating connectedness. Why is it so important; and furthermore, why does it seem so much more difficult to do in today's world than in the past?

McHenry

We were created to be in relationships with other people. Connectedness is a core need and component of wellness and health. Research indicates there are significant benefits from being in loving relationships and receiving loving touch. Connectedness is so central that babies who aren't held, die. In the penal system, the worst punishment for prisoners is to be put into solitary confinement. Connectedness came much more easily when individuals grew up, lived and died in the same communities that their grandparents had lived in and that future generations would live in as well. It was a slower time, with fewer distractions. Now we have sophisticated home entertainment systems and are able to shop and work from home. Many families are "too busy" to eat together and they no longer play games or even watch TV together because most have a television set, computer and telephone in their bedroom.

Furthermore, many no longer live close to extended families. Far too many of us don't even know the names of our neighbors, let alone what's happening in each other's lives. I distinctly remember being in college and seeing a walkman for the first time—I know I'm dating myself—but I remember thinking, "We're entering a world where we can tune each other out and nobody even has to hear each other's music." While we are extremely blessed to live in a society that offers so much, the price we pay for our mobility and the entertainment options we enjoy is that we're no longer naturally as connected as past generations. It's, therefore, imperative that we remember that connectedness is an important aspect of a healthy life and must be cultivated.

Wright

If someone wanted to develop safe and supportive relationships who should they let in; and what types of individuals should they screen out?

McHenry

First of all, it's very important to have good boundaries and to screen in order to develop safe and supportive relationships. When cultivating connectedness, find gentle truth tellers who don't hurt, humiliate or bash others. While it may be hard to hear the truth, it allows us to modify our behaviors so that we don't have broken relationships. Second, find people who like you for simply being you and who don't try to make you into someone else. Gravitate toward individuals who delight in you, these are the people who will flourish in your company and you in theirs! It's also important to cultivate relationships with individuals who make you laugh and bring you joy. Cultivate connectedness with those who will laugh and cry with you, and who will allow you to be angry without trying to fix or placate you. Cultivate connectedness with individuals with good boundaries, who are willing to listen to you, and that you respect and admire. Finally, screen out three types of individuals. The "drainers," individuals who suck the life out of you and rob your energy. The "takers," those who under-function, taking and taking from the relationship—resources, time, talent—without giving back. Most importantly, screen out "alligators," individuals who aren't safe and that willingly take a hunk of flesh when your back is turned. It's helpful to remember that the price of relationships, even with healthy individuals, is like the price of a rose. Bumping into thorns is inevitable if you get to know someone well over a span of time. It is sad, but true that everyone will at some point hurt or let you down. This is because we are human and are, therefore, destined to make mistakes. Let "roses" in, but screen out individuals who make snide and caustic remarks, as well as those who are emotionally or physically abusive. It is wisest to avoid individuals who willingly, for whatever reason, cause pain and damage another's soul.

Wright

From a wellness point of view, you talk about the need for individuals to also cultivate spirituality. What are the benefits of taking the time to develop spirituality? What happens when spirituality is ignored?

McHenry

The research on spirituality absolutely amazes me, David. When defining spiritual people as those who pray and attend church regularly, studies show that such individuals have lower blood pressure and are hospitalized less often than those who aren't spiritual. People with spirituality are also less likely to suffer depression; and when they do, they are more likely to recover, as well as, recover more quickly. Additionally, they report a stronger sense of well being, have better immune systems and recover more quickly from colds and illnesses than their non-spiritual counterparts. Furthermore, spiritual individuals experience less physical pain than those who are not. The fact that amazes me most is that spiritual individuals live eight years longer than their non-spiritual counterparts. I was just reading a study this morning by Dr. Lebron McBride, a physician suggesting that doctors begin asking patients about their spirituality so that they can include it more and more in the medical field.

In Western society, we've separated the body and the soul, but there's obviously a strong connection between the two. In addition to the health benefits, spirituality grounds people, as well as, provides meaning and significance. People with faith in God or in a higher power believe that someone more powerful than themselves is working on their behalf. Therefore they don't have to try to be God and waste unnecessary time and energy trying to control and be everything. Spirituality also guides behavior, which is speculated to be one of the reasons spiritual individuals live so much longer than others. Additionally, people who have ignored spirituality report that while it can be pushed aside for a very long time; feelings of emptiness persist. Unfortunately, a lot of people have been wounded by faith and by religiosity and in order for them to cultivate spirituality, they've got to go back and heal those wounds. As they've been wounded by imperfect people, I highly suggest they find healthier churches and individuals who extend grace and allow them the freedom to grow without being beaten down. When truth is searched for, it can be found, and the emptiness can be filled. Many have found *Toxic Faith*, by Stephen Arterburn and Jack Felton to be a very healing read.

Wright

You also focus on helping individuals access and utilize humor to maximize wellness and health. What does humor do for us; and will you share guidelines for appropriate vs. inappropriate humor?

McHenry

There's also a great deal of research about the benefits of humor. Humor eases our worries and frees us to move forward. It also provides hope, releases tension and aids in coping with life's stressors and illnesses. Humor has been shown to improve quality of life, increase circulation, aid the immune system and reduce pain. Furthermore, humor unites us, creates bonds and improves relationships. We live in a society that highly values humor and humorous people, and when we bring humor into relationships, we create an energizing force. There are many ways to cultivate a sense of humor beginning with simply looking for what's funny in life. Get out and watch people and observe yourself—I guarantee you'll find humor. I know I get tickled at what I do and what I see others doing. Watch funny movies and TV shows, read the funny pages, make funny faces in the mirror and tell jokes... I work on choosing laughter despite the pain and frustrations of the circumstances I encounter. The master at this, and the one who has most inspired me, is Steve Rizzo. His book, *Becoming a Humor Being* is fabulous. If you ever get the chance to see him, take it! He's absolutely hilarious and shares a powerful message about the need for, and benefits of, humor. He also addresses developing and utilizing humor in our lives.

Before we move on, I want to address your question concerning appropriate vs. inappropriate humor. Humor at the expense of an individual is always inappropriate, as is humor at the expense of a people group. While racial, ethnic or religious jokes may be funny and get a laugh, they wound and perpetuate negative stereotypes. While most in today's society are sophisticated enough to agree that it is inappropriate to tell ethnic or racial jokes, there are still two people groups that are the target of destructive humor; men and overweight individuals. My hope is that one day soon it will be as unacceptable to make fun of, demean, ridicule and tell jokes about these two groups as it is to tell racial jokes. The other inappropriate and destructive use of humor is using it to convey wounding messages. What I'm talking about are the "jabs" for which offenders blame the receiver for "not having a sense of humor." People know when they've been stung by inappropriate humor. It's helpful to know that such attacks are launched by individuals who instead of dealing with problems directly lurk about in the shadows waiting to zing unsuspecting individuals. Such attacks are strategic and destructive and reflect unresolved anger. Healthy individuals deal with their frustrations by directly addressing and working through problems, and therefore, have no need to "jab" others.

Wright

I've been doing training and speaking for the last 35-40 years; and it never ceases to amaze me what people learn and how they retain with humor. If you infuse humor in a training session, most people will get it. It's strange that humor is such a catalyst for learning. I also know in my life there have been some really terrible things that humor helped both me and my family to overcome.

McHenry

I love that you and your family have used humor to help overcome adversity. I also believe that the most gifted teachers and speakers are those who invite the audience to laugh; because appropriate humor lowers our defenses and opens us to learning. I'm glad you pointed that out because I line up with you exactly.

Wright

In my experience, I especially think they like the humor where I'm the butt of the joke. When it's all my fault and it's me that messed up. It amazes me what people remember.

McHenry

Many speakers, experts and executives are viewed as unapproachable. By laughing at our own foibles and inviting others to laugh with us, we instantly become authentic and congruent! When individuals combine humor and being real, people are drawn to them and what they have to say in an incredibly powerful way. No wonder you're so good at what you do!

Wright

Another key component of health and wellness is the development of healthy coping strategies. What unhealthy strategies would individuals do well to avoid; and on the flip side, what strategies are considered helpful?

McHenry

Unhealthy coping strategies are ways that people "zone" and "numb out" in order to avoid problems and unpleasant feelings. Engaging excessively in otherwise appropriate activities enables individuals to avoid dealing with what's really going on in their life such as broken relationships, unfulfilled hopes and dreams, unruly children, financial strains, tedious work or unemployment. Examples of unhealthy strategies include indulging in too much alcohol, television, food, gambling and sex. Workaholism and keeping busy are also problematic, even though they are socially acceptable and rewarded in our society. In short, pretty much any -ism or activity that allows individuals to "check out" and avoid having to face their problems, fears and feelings is an unhealthy coping mechanism. Regrettably, it's very common in our society for individuals to work all day and then watch television all evening. While it enables the individual to put off dealing with their problems, life and important relationships suffer. Spouses and children want, and need, "checked out" individuals to be an active part of their lives.

Additionally, the destructive effects of alcoholism, gambling addictions, sexual and pornography addictions and eating disorders wreck havoc with the individual and negatively impact the individuals in that person's life. What pushes something over into an unhealthy coping strategy is using it in excess. While it's okay to watch television and can even be a good way to feed an individual's humorous side, watching six hours of television a night and neglecting important relationships is problematic. Again, the key is balance. Unfortunately, individuals excessively engaging in unhealthy coping strategies are rarely able to discern balance. That's one of the reasons why it is so important to have, and to be willing to listen to, gentle truth tellers. As stress and problems are always going to be part of life, it's imperative that individuals cultivate healthy coping strategies. Examples of helpful and life improving strategies include journaling, exercising, eating healthy foods, cultivating quiet and solitude and slowing down long enough for the body to rest. Such activities have the added benefits of allowing individuals to think, figure out who they really are and develop increased insight and creativity. Society is so busy and offers so many distractions that it is generally necessary to make time to be still.

Over the past few years, I've chosen not to not work on Sundays and the benefit I've received is increased energy, efficiency and creativity throughout the week. Other healthy coping strategies that breath energy, resiliency and life into individuals include identifying and pursuing hopes and dreams. So is making time to do the things you love as an individual and as a family. My biggest love is downhill skiing. Being outside and flying down ski slopes makes me laugh with the sheer joy of living.

Therefore, I strategically budget time and money to ski. I consistently find that when I make time to rejuvenate my soul, I have increased energy and productivity. Lastly, learning to listen to the messages our bodies send is also part of healthy living and can significantly help avert injury. The body is finely tuned to provide messages through aches, pain and tiredness. When we override these messages, we risk causing serious damage. I don't want to give the impression that I only engage in healthy behaviors and always listen to the messages that my body sends. I don't, but the healthier I become, both mentally and physically, the more I improve. I still fight watching too much television, eating too much junk food and not getting enough exercise. Each of us struggles with one or more of these areas, but by developing increasingly healthy coping strategies, we can significantly improve our health and wellness.

Wright

Helping individuals identify and pursue their passions and dreams is also a passion of yours. Why is this critical to one's health and wellness? How do individuals go about doing it; and what are key passion killers?

McHenry

The reason I am so passionate about individuals pursuing their passions and dreams is because it allows them to fully live and utilize the gifts they've been given. In order for people to begin to pursue hopes and passions, they must first be able to envision that things can be different. I work with individuals and organizations to create healthy environments that enable them to see possibilities and unleash creative power. What isn't dreamed, isn't achieved! Once individuals and organizations are empowered to dream, transformation occurs! Unfortunately many individuals and organizations are wounded or have become resigned to existing in their current state. Many have been taught not to hope and or dream, because unfulfilled hopes and dreams can lead to disappointment and dashed hope.

My father always taught me that the price of being a dreamer is occasional pain and disappointment. He also regularly encouraged me to dream anyway because it is only when we dream that the possibility of achieving exists. I regularly shoot for the stars knowing that if I miss them, that I can usually catch the moon on my way back down. Have I been hurt and had dashed hopes and dreams? Absolutely, but I've also had incredible dreams come true. While there is never a guarantee, the risks are far outweighed by what I stand to gain by stepping out in faith and taking a chance. I love helping others begin to take the risk of hoping and dreaming, because it is only in risking that we find our passions.

In addition to taking risks, people wanting to live lives of passion and purpose must also avoid passion killers such as inauthenticity, having poor boundaries, failing to figure out and prioritize what's important and regularly engaging in unhealthy coping strategies. Unless we learn to spend our time, energy and resources judiciously, our dreams and passions fall by the wayside. In order to live at the highest level, we must work through our problems, fear and pain. Getting stuck in our comfort zone, pessimism, fear, restrictive thinking and believing "this is as good as it is going to get" also keep us from pursuing and reaching our dreams. When we chose to pursue our passions and to live emotionally, physically and spiritually healthy lives, we are able to face the future with a sense of well-being, excitement and hope.

Wright

Today, we've been talking to Dr. Sherene McHenry, an obvious expert in human relations. What a great conversation we've had. I sense she would be a perfect friend; and I believe that everyone reading this book will agree. I've learned a lot here today, and really appreciate you talking about passions. Probably more than any other single factor in my life, passion has made the biggest difference. Thank you so much for being with us on *Conversations on Health and Wellness*.

McHenry

Thanks for your kind words. I completely concur with you on passion, and have enjoyed our conversation immensely.

About The Author

Delivering highly understandable, usable and transferable knowledge with energy, heart and humor makes human relations expert, Dr. Sherene McHenry, a dynamic and captivating speaker with audiences around the world. Sherene's life has been one of challenge, adventure and achievement. She's skydived, flown solo and dined with a United States President. Over the past decade, Sherene has spoken to hundreds of audiences galvanizing them with real-life messages that inspire, enlighten and motivate. Dr. McHenry skillfully empowers businesses, organizations, couples and individuals to create genuine, reliable and trustworthy connections that maximize potential and create success.

Dr. Sherene McHenry, LPC
P.O. Box 1272
Mt. Pleasant, Michigan 48804
Phone: 989-779-7428
Fax: 989-772-0747
Email: info@ShereneMcHenry.com
www.ShereneMcHenry.com

Chapter 17

ANASTASIA L. TURCHETTA, RDH

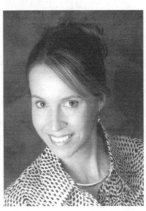

THE INTERVIEW

David E. Wright (Wright)

Today we are talking to Anastasia L. Turchetta, RDH. She has been a practicing clinical hygienist for 16 years, primarily on the east coast. Her degrees in dental assisting and dental hygiene were earned at Alleghany Community College in Cumberland, Maryland. She has written articles for both Contemporary Oral *Hygiene* and *Dental Practice Report.* She is a member of S.C.N., A.D.H.A., A.V.D.S., and N.S.A as well as president of Strategic Hygiene, which provides public presentations and consultations on incorporating the assisted hygiene program into dental practices. Anastasia, welcome to *Conversations on Health and Wellness*!

Anastasia L. Turchetta (Anastasia)

Thank you.

Wright

You know as I read your bio, I thought I was playing Scrabble. I have all of these letters that I have absolutely no idea what they mean. What is RDH?

Anastasia

Registered Dental Hygienist.

Wright

S.C.N.?

Anastasia

Speaking and Consulting Network.

Wright

A.D.H.A.?

Anastasia

American Dental Hygienists Association.

Wright

A.V.D.S.

Anastasia

American Veterinary Dental Society.

Wright

And I know what N.S.A. is. That's the National Speakers Association.

Anastasia

Correct!

Wright

So you can actually clean dogs' teeth?

Anastasia

Absolutely! I always take the opportunity to teach my pet-loving patients that their dogs and cats are susceptible to gum disease, just as we are. They need to know that they and their veterinarian are responsible for their pets' oral care. Although it is not a daily occurrence, my Siberian husky has her teeth routinely brushed and flossed. She will actually follow me into the bathroom when she hears the sound of my electric brush!

Wright

What causes dry mouth? And what products may or may not help dry mouth?

Anastasia

Dry mouth is very common and will most likely be detected during a dental visit. About 500 medications can produce xerostomia or dry mouth. Some medications include antidepressants, antianxiety, antihistamines, high blood pressure, antidiarrheals, muscle relaxants and antiparkinsonians. Other contributing factors may be radiation treatments to the head and neck area, Alzheimer's disease, stroke, smoking or chewing tobacco, snoring, breathing with your mouth open, diabetes, and autoimmune deficiencies such as Sjogren's syndrome. With Sjogren's syndrome, the immune system attacks a person's own body, mainly focusing on the salivary and tear glands. For more information pertaining to Sjogren's syndrome visit www.Sjogrens.org.

Our salivary glands will generally produce about three pints of saliva a day. Individuals who experience a decrease in saliva are susceptible to dental caries, sore mouth, difficulty in denture retention, chewing and swallowing, and recurrent oral yeast infections. Some try to alleviate the problem by drinking and/or eating products that contain sugar. Take note to identify what the main ingredients are in beverages as well as gum or mints. How would you determine if you have a dry mouth (xerostomia)? Take the "cracker" test. Chew a cracker without sipping water, if you have trouble with either swallowing or chewing the cracker you have xerostomia.

Our responsibility as dental professionals is to introduce products that manage the discomfort. For instance, Biotene, a product that may be offered within the dental practice or over the counter (OTC), offers a variety of salivary substitutes for patients such as toothpaste; alcohol free mouthwash, chewing gum and moisturizing gel. You may find this product at www.laclede.com. Rembrandt, known for their whitening products, also offer alcohol free mouthwashes, which may likewise be OTC or within the dental practice. For more information visit www.rembrandt.com. Professionally applied topical fluoride, whether a foam, gel, rinse or varnish is recommended to the patient during a preventative care appointment with the dental hygienist. Additional professional fluoride home care products may also be discussed at this time. Ask your dental hygienist for more information concerning the advancements in treating xerostomia.

Wright

Is gingivitis reversible?

Anastasia

Gingivitis precedes periodontal disease and is reversible if treated early. Gingivitis is defined as inflammation of the gum or soft tissue. Signs of gingivitis include swollen, tender, red gums that bleed easily when tooth brushing and flossing due to inadequate plaque removal. Hormonal changes, vitamin deficiencies, diabetes, drug influence, fungal or viral infections, blood disorders and immune-compromised disorders contribute to the cause of gingivitis. Most people tend to think that it's OK if your gums bleed, stating, "They've always bled." Because patients can't see the inflammation and many people are afraid to visit the dentist, people tend to put it off. I have enlightened those individuals with the following analogy, "A consultation with an urologist is warranted upon noticing blood in your urine; you are encouraged to do the same with your dentist regarding your bleeding gums."

Gingivitis is common in patients who receive orthodontic therapy, undergo assisted living care such as nursing homes, or are noncompliant toward their home care as well as preventative care appointments, which are routinely twice a year.

Treatment for gingivitis includes professional removal of both tartar and plaque by a dental hygienist. Depending upon the stage of gingivitis, it may be necessary to complete treatment in two appointments rendered by the dental hygienist. The hygienist first charts the inflamed areas in the mouth so they may be monitored in the future; then the hygienist reviews home care instructions such as brushing technique, interproximal plaque removal and mouth rinse, all of which should be performed daily.

Wright

What health problems have been linked with periodontal disease?

Anastasia

Periodontal disease has been linked to diabetes, heart disease, lung disease, and low birth weight or premature births in pregnant women.

It is estimated that 16 million Americans live with diabetes and approximately one-third are unaware that they have this disease. Patients who have diabetes must pay particular attention if they are diagnosed with periodontal disease, as it will become more difficult to control their blood sugar. For instance, I had a patient who was Type II diabetic, but he didn't know it. He had Type II periodontal disease. We had him coming in every three months; his home care was absolutely excellent, although we couldn't quite reach our goal for optimal oral health. He did not seem to fit the profile: he wasn't overweight, had no family history of diabetes, was under forty-five years of age, and he had his hypertension under control. About a year and a half later, he was diagnosed with diabetes when he attended a health fair at a local school. I have to wonder if the suppressed oral health was an early sign of diabetes. With his blood sugar levels under control, he is currently maintaining a four -month periodontal maintenance plan and reaping the rewards of a healthy oral environment.

Research has shown that women who have periodontal disease during their pregnancy are seven times more likely to have a baby pre-maturely in addition to a low birth weight. It would be advantageous for both medical and dental professionals to communicate with each other pertaining to prenatal care for their clients through educational pamphlets and/or programs.

As for the relationship linking both periodontal and lung disease, it has recently been discovered that oral bacteria found within periodontal pockets can be aspirated into the lungs causing an ailment such as pneumonia.

Wright

So tell me how nutrition plays a role in dentistry, or does it?

Anastasia

More now that ever, nutrition plays a role in our patients' oral health. When I was in college we had an assignment concerning nutritional counseling with our patients.

I thought, "Am I going to use this information in the real world?" Today, as you know, there are vending machines in the high schools, gyms, malls, etc. and parents are not able to monitor what their children are ingesting, nor how much of it. What was once an eight-ounce can, became twelve ounces and soon it's up to thirty-two ounces etc. We're seeing a lot of young children and teens with white spots along the gum line, which represent the start of cavities in the enamel, called decalcification. Soft drinks, sweet tea, fruit juices, chewing gum and mints are often the culprit. The following are examples of how nutrition plays a role in dentistry.

Parents should be advised of the type of beverage day-care centers are providing for their children. Some centers require the parents to furnish juice for what their children may drink during their stay. Recently I worked with a four-year-old girl whose teeth showed rampant decay. Many parents believe that baby teeth are not important, baby teeth are space maintainers for the permanent teeth. She should lose her last baby molar around the age of twelve. Her father explained what a normal day was like nutritionally for his daughter. She did not eat candy or sticky foods, but she was drinking several juice boxes a day.

It is essential for parents to have their children's teeth examined by a dentist by the age of 2 or 3 for several reasons. Benefits for the child include, determining if the child has early signs of caries, formulating a nutritional guide along with the parents, beginning professional applied fluoride options, and developing a routine preventative care regimen whether it be once or twice a year. A positive dental experience can be instilled early and last throughout the child's life.

Older people are at risk as well. People in nursing homes are generally on a soft food diet, which allows the food to stick to their teeth. Due to the fact that nursing homes are understaffed, oral health is not so much of a concern as bathing and changing each person. End result, the food lies on the teeth promoting either cavities or gingivitis.

Wright

I know my mother had Alzheimer's for fifteen years before she died, and in the later years it was almost impossible to take her to the dentist, as she wouldn't open her mouth. The dentist gave us little sticks with a sponge attached to it. Toothpaste was also on it. I used to brush her teeth with that, and she kind of enjoyed it.

Anastasia

I'm certain that she liked the clean feeling!

Wright

Dental care is really a serious problem in nursing homes.

Anastasia

It truly is, as most don't have an onsite facility or treatment room set up for dental equipment. Certain states now are starting to pass laws that enable dental hygienists to perform preventative care within the facility, which will benefit many patients.

During the dental visit, it is important to identify the occupation of each patient as this offers insight for the dental team to find a solution concerning the dental caries now present. For example, a truck driver or auto mechanic is more likely to be sipping soda throughout their workday. The dental hygienist recognizes the decalcification and asks the patient what type of beverage is preferred and how often. Gum and mints that aren't sugar free become a popular choice, especially with individuals who have quit smoking. Your enamel can only take so much of this acid attack before decalcification occurs eventually becoming weak, thus a cavity is formed.

Case in point, a teenager who previously had not developed dental caries presented some areas of decalcification at her preventative care appointment. Upon narrowing down the nutritional regimen, she admitted to chewing a certain brand of gum daily that was not sugar free. Frequency of intake was around five to eight sticks per day. She stated that this product gave her energy! I admit to trying the gum, alas, no added level of energy! She did not change her daily habit, and in spite of the fact, eventually developed dental caries on the decalcified teeth along the gum line, as well as in-between her teeth.

Wright

So is it the sugar in the soda?

Anastasia

Foods or beverages, containing starches, sugar or carbohydrates adhere to the tooth surface and weaken the enamel when not properly brushed and/or flossed off. In order to strengthen the enamel, fluoride treatments are required at least twice a year.

Dental caries and periodontal disease are caused by specific types of bacteria. Periodontal disease is originated via different types of bacteria. Interesting enough, whomever you were around when you were an infant introduced the bacteria or dental flora you have within the age of 6-30 months. For instance, an expecting mother who is a high caries risk may be recommended to chew gum containing xylitol, for prevention of introducing those specific bacteria to her baby. It is essential for expecting mothers to receive an assessment of caries or periodontal risk during their preventative care appointment with the dental hygienist.

Wright

It is very interesting. Are there tests available to detect oral cancer?

Anastasia

Currently, there are two tests available to dental practices, as oral cancer is something that you never think it's going to happen to you. Though, if detected early, it has a seventy-five percent cure rate.

One product is called Vizilite, made by Zila pharmaceuticals. The patient is to swish with the mouth rinse for thirty seconds; the lighting is dimmed to aid with illumination via a pen, which is activated to place in the patient's mouth. The cancerous cells will light up like a white t-shirt in black light. This test is convenient for patients, as they are able to receive a service within an environment they feel comfortable in. Once the dentist determines the outcome of the test, he or she may refer the patient to an oral surgeon for a biopsy. The second test is called Oral CDX and that is a brush biopsy made by CDx Laboratories. It looks like a toothpick with bristles, although when a sight looks very suspicious, you would rub the bristles into that area vigorously because you've got to get the cells onto the brush. Place in the test tube; send it off the lab, which will notify the dental practice within a few days whether it is positive or negative.

We've developed a definite relationship on trust and value with our patients. We know them better than their physicians probably know them, therefore, if we see anything, we can encourage them to get it taken care of. Most often patients do not go to the oral surgeon when referred for various reasons. By performing either test in office we can ease them into the next step in maintaining an overall healthy environment.

Wright

So what are the symptoms of oral cancer?

Anastasia

Symptoms of oral cancer ordinarily occur on the lip or tongue as a small pale colored area that is usually painless, though a burning sensation may develop later on. It may also be found on the palate, floor of the mouth and cheek lining. The National Cancer Institute calculates that 30,000 people will be diagnosed this year and of those, 8,000 will die. Although the exact cause is unknown, both cigarette and cigar smoking and smokeless tobacco are considered to be primary causes.

What I have personally noticed about oral cancer is, it's not very obvious. It could be a tiny red spot. It could be a tiny white spot. Here at the beach, Outer Banks of North Carolina, I have seen more oral cancer on the lip. Because of living at the beach, people who surf or fish may not be using sunscreens regularly.

Wright

Let's talk about services that we or I as a client should expect. What services should a patient receive during a preventative care appointment?

Anastasia

I believe that patients should not only expect the best possible care, but also receive it not matter what stage of life. Consider every question in this section a must have for each patient. A complete medical history review should be updated. It is important to ask each patient if there have been any changes in their health, such as surgeries, medications and herbals, since their last visit. Next, blood pressure is recorded and compared with previous reading. Normal reading is 120/80, a pre-hypertension category is determined when the reading is 120-139/80-89. For the most part we do see patients more than a physician, chiropractor or optician particularly with men. Keep in mind that blood pressure may be a little high if someone's a bit nervous about coming in for his or her dental appointment. If the blood pressure recording were alarmingly high, we would refer to the physician immediately. A pre-rinse is recommended to decrease the aerosol created during the appointment. Checking for any signs of oral cancer by wrapping the tongue in gauze and looking on both sides, feeling underneath the tongue for any lumps or bumps and involving the patient throughout the process promotes a higher level of awareness for each patient. A caries assessment, ranging from high to low risk, on each patient decides how cavity prone that individual is.

Wright

What is caries?

Anastasia

A dental term for a cavity or decay.

Anastasia

You should be asked if you get cold sores. Just because a patient doesn't have one at the time of their appointment, doesn't mean they do not suffer from it. There are products to offer which reduce the duration.

Concerns about your smile or anything in your mouth should be addressed at this time. It is an opportunity to introduce new esthetic treatments.

A periodontal assessment should be obtained, which is measuring the pocket depth around each tooth and recording them. One to three millimeters with no bleeding is healthy. Four millimeters and over with bleeding demands the attention of both dental hygienist and patient in formulating a successful plan according to the severity or stage of gum disease. For example, the best treatment option could entail quadrant scaling or deep scaling and placement of locally administered antibiotics provided within the dental practice or a referral to a periodontist, who specializes in gum disease.

Wright

So when you're recording these measurements, are you talking about bone loss?

Anastasia

Yes, we are looking for indications of bone loss, gingivitis, recession (gum shrinks back from tooth) and tooth mobility. Eighty percent of the population has some form of gum disease. These should be measured on a periodontal patient every three to four months and at least once a year for a routine patient.

Wright

What is malodor?

Anastasia

It's bad breath!

Wright

I used to call that something else. It was a great big long word for bad breath.

Anastasia

Halitosis!

Wright

So how can a dental hygienist help with bad breath then?

Anastasia

There is a reason it has been called dog breath! As a dental hygienist, I am able to tactfully inform the patient by asking if they have noticed an aroma upon brushing or flossing. Obvious causes are food, beverages, tobacco smoking, throat infection, alcohol and sinusitis. What patients don't realize is that poor dental hygiene, gingivitis; uncontrolled periodontal disease and abscessed teeth are most likely the reason.

A dry mouth may also be associated with halitosis. The dental hygienist now must wonder why does this person have a dry mouth. Or why are they experiencing bad breath? Could it be related? So again, if it's related, you want to stay away from your alcohol mouth rinses. Oral hygiene products such as Breath RX, an alcohol free mouth rinse whose active ingredient in it is Zytex, target the volatile sulfur compounds which are main contributors to bad breath. For more information www.discusdental.com

Wright

Well, alcohol is a drying agent, isn't it?

Anastasia

Yes. Those individuals who are not taking any medication or experiencing xerostomia, products such as Listerine are wonderful. We've got to look at the medical history to observe medications as discussed above. Your dental hygienist can guide you as to what additional alcohol free products would best serve their needs.

Some individuals are not aware of the importance in brushing their tongue. Not everyone develops a buildup on his or her tongue, but many do. For example, when you drink coffee, a coating forms on the tongue afterwards; bacteria feed on the coating and create bad breath.

Wright

My dental hygienist told me once I was grown to brush my tongue, although I wish she had told me when I was in high school. I said, " I'm not going to brush my tongue." She said, "Well, if you don't you'll have halitosis."

Anastasia

It's true. This should be introduced in all hygiene appointments not matter what your age, as this may have an effect on one's self esteem.

Wright

What herbals could affect my dental visit?

Anastasia

It's very important to ask about herbals when the updating the patient's health history, as some are anti-coagulants. The result is an increase in bleeding and delayed healing that is not anticipated for certain dental treatment, i.e. periodontal therapy, implants, extractions. Granted, the daily dosage of these herbals should be considered as well as adverse effects from both prescription and over the counter medication the patient is currently receiving. Some of the herbals that are anti-coagulants are cat's claw, dong-quai, feverfew, evening primrose, garlic, ginger, ginkgo biloba, ginseng (Siberian form), green tea, and horse chestnut.

Two herbals that affect local anesthetic - particularly - epinephrine are ephedra and yohimbe. Both will increase blood pressure.

Wright

How does malocclusion relate to my health?

Anastasia

Malocclusion—crowded teeth, or misarranged teeth—is the most common reason that we would refer to an orthodontist. Very few people naturally have a beautiful smile. When the teeth are crowded, it is tougher for the individual to clean; therefore there is more risk for periodontal disease and tooth decay. Treatment can relieve symptoms of TMJ disorder (Temporal Mandibular Joint). It is important for our teeth to be aligned as the upper teeth keep the cheeks and lips from being bitten and the lower teeth protect the tongue. In addition, you will notice an abnormal appearance of the face thus affecting one's self esteem. Watch extreme makeover and relish that individual's constant smile!

Even though malocclusion is often hereditary, habits such as thumbsucking, tongue thrusting and pacifier use beyond the age of four can change the shape of the jaw.

Depending upon the severity of crowding determines the length of time it will take to successfully treat the patient. Tooth extractions and jaw surgery may be required before orthodontic therapy. Discuss advances in orthodontics such as Invisalign, a clear alternative to traditional brackets.

There are three types of malocclusion.

- Type 1 malocclusion is the most common. The bite is normal, however, the teeth are crowded.
- Type 2 malocclusion is an overbite. The upper jaw projects over lower jaw.
- Type 3 malocclusion is an underbite. The lower jaw protrudes forward.

Wright

It's fascinating. How may assisted hygiene improve care provided to you as a patient? And what is assisted hygiene?

Anastasia

Assisted hygiene is defined as one dental hygienist working out of two treatment rooms with a designated dental assistant. So together, they provide unsurpassed care for that patient. You now have two care providers per patient. If a dentist were to work out of one room like a hygienist has been doing for years, you'd have to ask him or her how long would they stay in dentistry.

This is such an exciting time in dentistry due to the technological advances available. By adding a very valued team member, being a dental assistant, we are able to increase that level of care. For instance, recording blood pressure, pre-rinsing, utilizing the intra-oral camera and DIAGNOdent (a caries detection laser), applying desensitizing agents, updating x-rays, explaining an oral hygiene product for home care, clarifying treatment recommended, introducing sports guards or Toothprints (a wafer-like product which contains the child's bit registration and DNA for identification) to children and parents, comparing options for whitening, etc. make the visit easier and educational for them.

Four-handed dentistry is both quicker and more comfortable for patients. With children, we're able to place sealants at that visit versus reschedule them. If someone is interested in whitening, the dental assistant is able to get impressions for the take home tray system and the patient only has to come back once versus twice. When performing a quadrant scaling for a periodontal patient, the task of utilizing an ultrasonic instruments and placing locally administered antibiotics or antimicrobials is improved for both patient and dental hygienist on account of the dental assistant.

Assisted hygiene adds value because that's what's lacking a lot. Patient's attitudes reflect that it's just a cleaning. When you have two people who are excited about dentistry working with you, asking questions and performing services that may otherwise be passed over, it does create a value for that appointment; therefore, patients are less likely to cancel. They are able to accept and own what's going on in their mouth, which relates to their total health. Patients prefer assisted hygiene. It is more patient centered. One person can't perform or introduce each new area of dentistry to the patient. It does take two!

Wright

When I go to my dental hygienist and I leave the building, my first inclination is run my tongue all over my mouth to see what happened. Everything is just so clean.

Anastasia

It feels so slick and refreshing!

Wright

Well, what an interesting conversation. I'm going to go right out and brush my tongue and scrape it, you know.

Anastasia

Don't forget to floss, toothpick or water pik!

Wright

That's right and floss. I remember back many years ago, a famous dentist who then turned in to be a famous speaker, was telling the story about the lady that was complaining, "Well, I don't have to floss all my teeth, do I?" And he responded, "No, just the ones you want to keep."

Anastasia

I've heard that! I tell patients, " I have two words for you—floss daily." An analogy I have used; imagine if you brushed your teeth as often as you flossed what would you teeth feel like? Due to our busy lives, it is helpful to give tips for developing the habit of flossing, such as, keeping the floss near your computer. Most likely you're going to be downloading pictures to send or receive and it takes a few moments to do that. While you're waiting, you can floss!

Wright

That's right! Today we have been talking to Anastasia Turchetta. She is a registered dental hygienist. She's president of Strategic Hygiene, which provides public presentations and consultations on incorporating the assistant hygiene program into dental practices. We really do appreciate you spending this much time with us on *Conversations on Health and Wellness*. Thank you so much for your time.

Anastasia

Thank you. It has been my pleasure.

About The Author

Anastasia conducts seminars and consultations to practices and organizations which present a fresh approach in accomplishing optimum patient care via her expertise with assisted hygiene, passive income centers and pet dentistry. She is an independent sales representative for Viroxyn, a cold sore product. She is currently working on her next book where she resides in the Outer Banks, NC.

Anastasia L. Turchetta, RDH

Strategic Hygiene

PO Box 7656

Kill Devil Hills, North Carolina 27948

Phone: 252-202-9319

Fax: 252-441-5243

Email: strategichygiene@aol.com

www.strategichygiene.com